Nursing Ethics

For Hospital and Private Use

By Isabel Adams Hampton Robb

Graduate of the New York Training School for Nurses attached to Bellevue Hospital; late Superintendent of Nurses and Principal of the Training School for Nurses, Johns Hopkins Hospital Baltimore. Md.: late Superintendent of Nurses. Illinois Training School for Nurses. Chicago, Illinois; Member of the Board of Lady Managers Lakeside Hospital, Cleveland, Ohio: Honorary Member of the Matrons' Council, London. England.

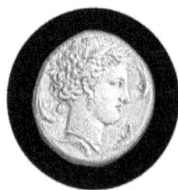

PANTIANOS
CLASSICS

Published by Pantianos Classics

ISBN-13: 978-1-78987-473-0

First published in 1900

Contents

Chapter One - Introductory Chapter 5

Chapter Two - Nursing as a Profession 10

Chapter Three - Qualifications 18

Chapter Four - The Probationer 23

Chapter Five - The Junior Nurse 30

Chapter Six - Health - The General Care of the Body 41

Chapter Seven - Uniform - Dress - Economy 51

Chapter Eight - Night-Duty 57

Chapter Nine - The Senior Nurse 63

Chapter Ten - The Head-Nurse 69

Chapter Eleven - The Graduate Nurse - Private Duty 79

Chapter Twelve - The Case of the Patient 95

All things whatsoever ye would that men should do to you, do ye even so to them. — Matthew vii, 12.

"Oh may I join the choir invisible
Of those immortal dead who live again
In minds made better by their presence — live
In pulses stirred to generosity,
In deeds of daring rectitude, in scorn
For miserable aims that end with self,
In thoughts sublime that pierce the night-like stars
And with their mild persistence urge men's search.
To vaster issues...May I reach
That purest heaven, be to other souls
The cup of strength in some great agony,
Enkindle generous ardour, feed pure love,
Beget the smiles that have no cruelty —
Be the sweet presence of a good diffused.
And in diffusion ever more intense.
So shall I join the choir invisible,
Whose music is the gladness of the world."

GEORGE ELIOT.

Chapter One - Introductory Chapter

If it were possible to bring together, from North, South, East and West all the trained nurses of the present time to be reviewed and to have judgment passed upon them, we should have before us a body not of conscripts but of volunteers, each of whom occupies her position in the ranks of her own free will and accord. At first no doubt we should be impressed with the magnitude of their numbers, and with the general good effect presented by their forces. But when we came to concentrate our attention upon each regiment, as it were, and upon each individual in that regiment, we should be struck with some not altogether pleasant incongruities. We should notice a certain lack of harmony in methods of drill, in deportment, in discipline, in uniform and in other minor details. As a body they do not always move in step; they are sometimes out of line, and some are inclined to straggle. We then glance at the officers for an explanation, but we find that they too are not always in harmony, though perhaps more so than are those in the ranks; still it is very apparent that each woman is a law unto herself in the matter of outer equipments at least, and we may notice in passing that her gaze seems to be largely concentrated upon her own particular regiment without a proper regard as to the manner in which its manoeuvres or actions may affect those in front, behind or on either side. We turn our attention again to the ranks and take notice of the individual members, but only here and there do we find an opportunity for a really favorable criticism. Nevertheless, now and again, our eyes are attracted to one who always stands at attention, constantly observant that she is in line, not elbowing, keeping her place indeed, but always with a due regard to those about her. She is alert, active, erect, well disciplined, yet withal of a modest demeanor and bearing. Her face tells the story for her that she has either brought from the outset into this work a mind and body well taught and self-disciplined, or else that she has been long in the ranks and under fire many times, and in the course of the struggle has attained an experience that always serves to tell her on the instant the difference between right and wrong — what to do and what not to do. And at the end we naturally turn to the officers and ask: "Why should there be this lack of harmony in our nursing ranks, this carelessness in regard to details, this evident overlooking of little things, that mean so much in the aggregate and when we are brought face to face with them? How is it that only here and there we find one approaching the ideal nurse, and why is it that even the officers are very little better than the rank and file in these respects?" And the answer is that we have just reviewed a body of women, enlisted in the same profession and under the same obligations, but in whose development no generally recognized ethical laws have had a part. By this it is not meant that trained nurses have lived thus far beyond the pale of ethics, but that, generally speaking, as members of one profession, they have been without an adopted code, the exceptions being in the case of isolated schools or alumnae associations. Any ideas of special moral responsibilities have been vague and indefinite to the many, while the few have evolved them for themselves as a result of observation and experience. Now, however, not only as individuals, but as a profession, we are beginning to feel an increasing necessity for some such definite moral force or laws that shall bind us more closely together in this work of nursing, and that will bring us into more uniform and harmonious relations. I know of no other body of workers outside of physicians who need just such strength and stimulus as come from unity of purpose than do trained nurses, accustomed as they must become to deal with all sorts and conditions of men and circumstances. My purpose in the following chapters is not to attempt to formulate or even to suggest anything in the way of a formal code of ethics, but rather to consider briefly the nature of ethical laws and try to determine in what ways they may be made to have a practical bearing upon a nurse's duties and actions. I hope that what I shall say may be found useful as a text or basis upon which each superintendent of nurses may enlarge according to her knowledge and experience. I am convinced that many a woman's success, either as a pupil or a graduate nurse, is wrecked, not for lack of knowing how to do her work well, but from her ignorance or neglect of the practical application of the ethical side of her profession. Even where the ethical traditions of her school have been good and the teaching of ethical principles has not been neglected, I have known nurses — thoroughly well trained in other respects — to go out into private practice and commit the most flagrant breaches in the ethics and etiquette of their work. Perhaps, then, something that may be said may commend itself also to the graduate nurses, who possibly by reason of inexperience have not taken thought or time to reason out for themselves the underlying principles that ought to govern them in their professional life; certainly if they will quietly sit down, read, weigh and digest the various details of the subject, they cannot fail to reap some benefit. To those who have already reached the noonday of experience and have walked with senses alert and receptive, this dwelling upon details is perhaps not so necessary; indeed from the rich fullness of our several experiences — from what we have learned from our failures as well as from our successes — should come the formulated code of ethics, which should serve for the younger travellers in the guild as finger-posts along their nursing career to guide and encourage them at the crossways of purposes, until in the fullness of time they reach this knowledge for themselves. For though it be agreed that experience must ever remain our best teacher and guide, it would seem' that a sufficiency of it sometimes comes too late and that for the beginner her teachings can be to a certain extent supplied meanwhile by those she has already taught.

By *ethics* is meant the science that treats of human actions from a standpoint of right and wrong. It teaches men the practice of the duties of human life and the reasons for what they should do and for what they should leave undone. These duties are moral and relate more especially to the private and social relations of men; in course of time these regulations come to be regarded as expressing the received and customary sentiments concerning right and the duty between man and man, and their acceptance, therefore, implies free agency. Such moral duties differ from the positive duties in that they arise out of the nature of the case, while positive duties, on the other hand, are laid down by extraneous command.

In accepting such rules or laws one becomes subject to a principle or duty and is in honor bound to try and do what is right. This capability of discriminating between right and wrong is based on a knowledge of human nature and of the various relations in which man as a moral or social being is or may be placed. Our actions thus become directed by the mind.

The necessity for such moral rules of life being obvious, we find certain unwritten moral laws or rules of life which have been adopted by man in his relations to himself and to mankind in general and which are as strong as life itself. As human beings become formed into societies, guilds or crafts, these, besides following the broad, general moral laws, adopt certain regulations which morally are binding upon each member, although they may have no legal weight. These moral laws are necessary for the honor, integrity and the holding together of such societies and for their higher development.

We are all familiar with the saying "There is honor among thieves." I only quote it as a reminder that no matter how low in the social scale human beings may fall they still preserve some remnant of feeling with regard to the force of these moral laws. Since, then, codes of ethics must exist for all men and for all ages, in considering them in connection with our own profession of nursing we do but follow in the footsteps of mankind In general. The rules of conduct adapted to the many diverse circumstances attending the nursing of the sick institute *nursing ethics*.

In addition to ethics we employ another term to designate something which has a wide significance in connection with society at large and with particular guilds of associations. *Etiquette,* speaking broadly, means a form of behavior or manners expressly or tacitly required on particular occasions. It makes up the code of polite life and includes forms of ceremony to be observed, so that we invariably find in societies that a certain etiquette is required and observed either tacitly or by express agreement. Dr. Austin Flint expresses the distinction between medical ethics and medical etiquette as follows: "The former rules have a moral weight, while etiquette, on the other hand, consists of forms to be observed in professional intercourse and are conventional.

At the graduating exercises of almost every training school the physician who usually makes the address to the nurses, often feels it incumbent upon him to spend the hour in laying down rules and giving good ethical advice to those who are graduating. Not that he wishes to be officious in so doing, but he knows full well how far the fulfilment or neglect of such advice will go to make or mar the future success and work of the graduate nurse. At the same time he is probably aware that perhaps sufficient emphasis has not been laid upon the important during the years of training. Unfortunately, it is to be feared that his good advice will bear but little fruit if the teaching of these principles is left until this final hour. Instruction in the science of ethics and the rules of etiquette should be commenced from the moment the pupil-nurse enters a hospital, and from the very beginning of her term of probation. It should go hand in hand with the training in the theory and practice of nursing, otherwise the pupil will fail to realize its proper degree of importance and thus much benefit will be lost to her. Such instruction should be practical and systematic, beginning with the moral laws and rules she will need first to put in practice, and progressively leading up to an appreciation of her greater and higher obligations to herself, to her profession and to humanity. And no rule laid down or law required or taught but should bear with it the reason why, set forth simply and clearly. This systematic instruction should come largely from the superintendent herself, and should never or seldom be relegated primarily to any of the various members of her staff of head-nurses or assistants, although these by example and precept should never fail to emphasize this part of the training. Such teaching should have the extra force that it would receive coming from the head of the school and from her broader knowledge and experience. It seems to me that we have in days gone by thought too lightly of this branch of instruction in the making of nurses. For women engaged in almost any other class of work this special teaching might not seem so necessary; but to the nurse it is all important, for although she may be most thorough and skillful in all that pertains to the practical part of nursing, let her go into a family and omit or transgress some tittle of professional or social etiquette and all her practical knowledge will be of little value to her. On the other hand, given a nurse equipped with the tactful and common sense knowledge of the ethics and etiquette of her work, added to a thorough practical knowledge of nursing, and her future success is assured. The question will never be asked of her: Why cannot she get and keep patients? for she will always be in demand.

Heretofore, I fear we have done as much harm as good in the little we have tried to teach by the manner of teaching. Relegated to the head-nurse or her successive assistants, the senior or junior nurses, for instruction on these all-important points, the probationer has had rules and forms, sometimes contradictory, thrown at her head, so to speak, at divers times, and in a variety of fashions. What wonder then if she comes to regard all as rules to be avoided or broken at will, to be observed as little as possible; and furthermore, what wonder if our nurses leave us with no higher ideals or standards than those which we too often find among them. To be sure the argument is plausible that we are dealing with grown women, with habits already formed. Nevertheless, it would seem that two, or, better still, three years of systematic reasoning over and observing and testing certain forms of conduct must have a stronger influence for good than our hitherto unsystematic methods have given us. Provided with thorough instruction in this subject, when a nurse leaves her school, she will be ready to accept the more definitely formulated code of ethics and etiquette that are to henceforth govern her; if she then errs she does so wilfully. To digress for one moment. This point again emphasizes the importance of special instruction and qualifications for those nurses who look forward to becoming teachers and principals in training schools. Without certain definite and uniform requirements for our teachers we can no more look for uniformity in our ethics and etiquette than we can hope to attain it in our methods of teaching.

Perhaps at first glance it might be thought that this subject would require not more than two or three lectures or talks at the most and that our full duty would then be done. Let us consider what are some of these subjects that come under the heads of ethics and etiquette and then see how much time they should cover. In the first place we have hospital etiquette, with its various subdivisions as to duties, forms to be observed, discipline and kindred subjects; together with the similarities and distinctions between etiquette as suited to the hospital and to private practice. Next we have the ethical subjects, as for example, the importance and duty of systematically acquiring knowledge pertaining to our work and the methods to be employed; the care of the nurse's own health as a factor in doing good work and benefiting her patients and how this should be provided for; the scope and limitation of her professional authority; her personality as to cleanliness, manners, politeness; the significance and importance of her uniform, and other minor details.

The consideration of the development and application of the various selfs — self-reliance, self-restraint, self-possession, and many others — would by themselves occupy one lecture. Then come kindred topics such as tact, the proper manner of employing sympathy, sentiment, conversation, and the cultivation of the character-building virtues — patience, gentleness, cheerfulness, good temper — and their effect. Not a few hours might be taken up with the consideration of the ways and means of acquiring habits of exactness, truthfulness, method and order, vigilance and observation; finally, there are problems connected with remuneration and professional engagements and responsibilities. All such subjects as these should be fully considered by the teacher for the instruction of her pupils and as a help to them in realizing the practical application of the ethical principles involved in nursing. The dwelling upon them more in detail is an absolute necessity; and without it we can never hope to present to the public a profession in which harmony, uniformity and method are to be found, or to finally evolve a code of nursing ethics that will be of a thoroughly practical nature, one that we may be able to carry into our everyday lives and work, stimulating us to live for what is noble and best in each of us and developing a strength of character upon which a sick world may lean.

When writing my text-book on "The Principles and Practice of Nursing" I was constantly tempted to digress from the purely practical subjects in order to dwell at length upon the ethical side of our profession. As I went on, however, it soon became clear to me that the adoption of such a plan would result in an insufficient exposition of either side of nursing. I therefore decided to add a chapter at the end of the book. But by the time that this was only partially written I had become convinced that the subject needed on my own part much more extended observation and thought. Since that time my opportunities have been unusually good for judging of the importance of nursing ethics and for noting our lamentable deficiencies in this respect Finally, I resolved to undertake the task of writing upon the subject more in detail, in the hope that any suggestions I might be able to make might be the means of concentrating the attention of nurses upon this feature of their work and might afford them some encouragement to give to ethics more study and thereby bring them more prominently into their practical work. Only rarely does one hear criticisms directed against the purely practical work of a nurse; on the other hand the ethical side is being constantly attacked and too frequently, I fear, with sufficient cause. No one knows better than I do the splendid devotion and efforts that nurses as a body have shown and are showing every day in their efforts to raise the standard of nursing, but it requires the individual devotion to secure success and it is my confidence in our ultimate success and my faith in the women who are nurses that has encouraged me to go on with the subject, upon which I first began to write three years ago. The present introductory chapter appeared among the papers read at the Nurses' Exhibition in New York in 1897, but until the present year my spare time was so fully occupied with other nursing affairs that I was unable to make further progress. That the treatment of the subject is faulty and imperfect and that the half is not told, I am only too well aware. Nevertheless, such as they are, these pages are offered as the expression of a sincere desire on the part of a senior nurse to help the young ones, who come after her, to avoid the pitfalls that she would have been only too glad to have had pointed out to her and the knowing and understanding of which would not only have made her path easier, but would also have rendered her work more effective.

Chapter Two - Nursing as a Profession

That you may better understand the conditions now existing in the hospital and nursing world, I shall first briefly sketch some of the devious ways by which modern nursing has come to its present status, worthy to be ranked as an art and a profession. A full consideration of the entire range of this subject would far exceed the possibilities of a single chapter. The ancient history of hospitals and their methods of dealing with their sick both before and during the early days of Christianity would by itself afford abundant material for an interesting volume, while a second might deal with the rise and growth of the multitudes of monasteries and religious sisterhoods, which began in the middle ages and have lasted down to our own times. But although these events are full of intense interest from a historical standpoint, they had little to do in leading up to the present methods in hospitals and nursing. Only it may be remembered that one founder, among the many, seems to have spoken with prophetic voice of things to come when he ordained for the Sisters of Mercy of St. Vincent de Paul: "They shall have no monasteries but the house of the sick, no cells but a hired room, no cloisters but the streets of the town and the wards of the hospital, no inclosure but obedience, and for convent bars only the fear of God; for a veil they shall have a holy and perfect modesty; and while they keep themselves from the infection of vice they shall sow the seeds of virtue wherever they turn their steps." Hundreds of years have passed since those words were spoken, but they perfectly picture the ideals of the sisterhood of trained nurses at the close of the nineteenth century. And what more beautiful inspiration need a woman have to join forces to make such ideals daily facts?

Let us, then, leave nursing with its ancient and medieval conditions and confine ourselves to a consideration of what has been done during the last hundred years. It would seem that the first quarter of the century found a condition of affairs that in point of degradation could hardly be conceived possible. The hospitals stood for all that was bad; they were lazar-houses not only of physical horrors, but also of moral iniquity; the nursing was relegated to those among women who were not considered of sufficient respectability to be entrusted with the most menial of domestic work, and whose moral turpitude was equalled only by their incompetence. But during these years there were born into the world four people who lived to bring light into dark places and who by example and precept brought about a revolution. There is no need for me to speak to you at length of Elizabeth Fry and her work in prisons and hospitals, of Charles Dickens and his inimitable writings, of Pastor Fleidner, the founder of the order of German Deaconesses, and last but not least, of our own beloved Miss Nightingale. Their names will live forever in our hearts and in the hearts of those who come after us.

With the last two, however, we have more to do just now, since they were practically the founders of the present system of nursing the sick. Theodor Fleidner was born in the year 1800, in the small village of Eppstein on the frontiers of Hesse and Nassau, where his father was the parish clergyman. At the age of 20 he himself became the pastor of the little town of Kaiserwerth on the Rhine, which has become famous for all time on account of the great work which he established there. On an income of $125 a year he managed not only to exist, but also to help his parishioners, who were in a condition of extreme poverty, and a prey to dirt and disease. Before he had lived there very long, even this income became diminished owing to the failure of the velvet manufactories which supplied work to most of his parishioners. As a result he was obliged to cast about to save his church and help his neighbors in their distress, and with this object in view he made journeys through Germany, Holland and England, pleading his cause with more or less success. But from these journeys was realized something of far more value than the money he raised. He brought back with him an experience and knowledge of what was being done in other countries in the way of charitable enterprise. While in England he encountered Elizabeth Fry, and as a result his attention became directed towards prison reform. On his return to Germany, he set about founding an asylum for discharged women prisoners and appealed to Christian womanhood to support him in his work. In 1833 the first woman prisoner, who later became the first deaconess, arrived in Kaiserwerth. At the same time Fleidner founded his hospital, beginning with a single patient. But even for this one patient a nurse was necessary. The recognition of this need led to the founding, or rather the reviving of the order of Deaconesses, which the church in its early days had established as necessary to its successful working, but which as time went on had been allowed to disappear. How the improvements thus instituted by Pastor Fleidner have advanced still further until they have spread all over the world, I need not mention in detail. I will only refer to the way in which his work was brought into direct connection with the system of modern nursing through Florence Nightingale, the founder and heroine of hospital nursing as it now exists and the patron saint of nurses.

Miss Nightingale was born at Florence, Italy, in 1820, her parents being English gentle people of influence and wealth. A natural philanthropist, while still a very young woman, she was stirred, in her inmost soul by the deplorable care given to the sick both inside and outside of hospitals. Urged on by an intense desire to do something towards removing this reproach to the intelligence and humanity of the nineteenth century, she left her home and went from place to place in Europe examining the different systems employed in the various countries and comparing one with the other. As the fruit of these pilgrimages we have her book entitled "Notes on Hospitals" — rich in suggestions for practical reforms. In these she laid particular stress upon sanitary construction in hospitals, and to what she then wrote we owe the attention that from that time on began to be devoted to sanitation and hygiene, the perfection of which we now find in new hospitals the world over. But Miss Nightingale recognized that in order to do effective work in bettering matters, it was necessary to supplement her theoretical knowledge by a practical acquaintance with the subject. As the result of several months spent at Kaiserwerth on two different occasions, she was able to write: "I at once recognized what I had so long sought — a spirit of devotion, of order and unity of purpose. It was impossible not to be impressed with the air of purity and deep, unaffected piety which pervaded the whole place; and yet there was no asceticism; it was the world, and yet not the world in the ordinary sense of the word. There was the mother, Madame Fleidner, the pastor's wife, mother of his large family, laying no claim to the dignity of "Lady Supe-rior," but a plain Christian woman, who had not found the duties of wife and mother incompatible with spiritual cares, when both alike were exercised under one and the same guide and director, her husband. There were the young deaconesses with their intelligent animated countenances, no mere instruments yielding a blind and passive obedience, but voluntary and en-lightened agents, obeying, on conviction, an inward principle."

In 1849 Miss Nightingale enrolled herself as a voluntary nurse in this es-tablishment, and thus became practically acquainted with the various forms of disease and a good system of nursing. It seems need-less to recapitulate here what the world owes to her for her work during the Crimean war. How she sped is a matter of universal knowledge. Upon her return to England a grateful English public placed at her disposal contributions to the amount of 50,000 pounds sterling. With this fund she founded the Nightingale Training School for Nurses, the first of its kind, so soon to be duplicated in the United Kingdom and thence throughout the world. In 1873 Sister Helen, a Nightin-gale Sister or Trained Nurse, came over to America and started the New York Training School for Nurses in connection with Bellevue Hospital, in the City of New York. Somewhat later in the same year similar schools were opened in New Haven and Boston.

The conditions existing in hospitals at that time in this country were very little, if at all, better than those abroad, and one would have supposed that a respectable, intelligent class of women, offering themselves for hospital work, would have been received with open arms. Unfortunately, such was not the case. Months or years of hard physical and mental work, before she could obtain her certificate, represented but a small part of the struggle through which, a quarter of a century ago, or even less, a woman had to pass before she could establish her claim to share in hospital work as a trained nurse. It was a long while, indeed, before even the medical profession as a body regarded her with favor. But after physicians had once begun to realize that with trained nursing it was possible to have their orders intelligently carried out, that chaos and dirt gave way to order and cleanliness, that the percentage of deaths decreased and of recoveries increased; lastly, when once for all they had learned to recognize the fact that their own particular province was in no danger of invasion, they finally accorded to the trained nurse her professional recognition.

The history of the education of the people at large upon this point forms an interesting chapter in sociology. The care — or perhaps we might say the criminal negligence — accorded to poor patients in hospitals in days gone by had made the name "hospital" a by-word and a term of reproach, which is not yet wholly eradicated from the minds of the ignorant and even of those who should be better informed. The prevailing type of attendants upon the sick in the early years of the century had accustomed people to regard paid nurses as self-seeking menials, engaged in something far lower than domestic work, and whose only object was to benefit by others' misfortunes at the least expenditure of care and trouble on their own part. It is true that in all ages we have had noble women who devoted their whole life to their religion and to the care of the sick, and hence there have existed at all times another class of nurses, many of noble birth, all of noble souls, whose memory must ever be held in respect and honor. But here again too often the will was taken for the deed. It was apparently only necessary to wish to take proper care of the sick and to proceed at once to do so. Hence resulted a sad waste of much well-meant energy and too little progress so far as the welfare of the sick was concerned. But the views of the people were gradually growing broader. From regarding nursing the sick as an occupation for paid menials, or as a service of sacrifice and self-abnegation, to be shrouded in the garments of a religious sisterhood, they gradually reached the idea that widows and un-married women of a certain age and experience might also find here a field of work. But to a public educated up to even this pitch it still came as a shock to find respectable women — young and unmarried — willing to give up two years of their life in a hospital to learn how to take care of the sick and to claim their right to establish the profession of trained nursing. Nevertheless, despite prejudices, institutions for instruction in nursing were established which were educational as well as humanitarian in their principles.

Unfortunately at first the number of competent women who were willing to enter training schools was somewhat limited and these* institutions were, therefore, obliged to offer a certain amount of monetary inducement in order to secure pupils in sufficient numbers. This fact is much to be regretted, since it has emphasized the commercial and the manual side at the expense of the educational standpoint of such schools.

The movement, once started, spread with great rapidity. Schools grew up on all sides, and as might have been expected, the competition for pupils was for a time so great that educational requirements for admission were kept unduly low. This feature has proved detrimental to the best interests of nurs-ing in many ways. For the average nurse a preliminary education little be-yond that furnished by the public schools has been demanded. It is true that in the better schools preference is given to applicants of superior education and cultivation and that not a few trained nurses are women of considerable attainments. But this low standard of requirement has increased the tenden-cy of the public to regard the skill of the trained nurse as largely mechanical and her work as almost wholly manual, affording but little scope for a trained intellect. Again, it must be confessed that much has been done to justify this opinion by the appallingly long hours of practical work which have been and are still required, in too many hospitals, of the pupil-nurse. Certainly, after 9 or sometimes 12 or 13 hours spent in the wards, little time and still less brain power is left for theoretical study, and even to the most intelligent and earnest mind fatigue is almost the only sensation left.

The question as to the social status of the trained nurse is also of interest. At one time it required not a little moral courage on the part of a refined woman to take up nursing. Her position had to be maintained day and night under the constant, vigilant, and not always friendly, criticism of the free ward patients, whose verdict, like that of the gallery gods judging an artist on the stage, carried weight not only in the hospital, but also in the slums of the city whence the majority of her patients were drawn. For it is the poorest patients who decide in part whether others will avail themselves of the benefits of the hospital; and every nurse should feel that with her rests to a great extent the power of such institutions to do the greatest good to the greatest number. Again, it was a long time before the young house physician could bring himself to understand that the trained nurse was there as his assistant and not as his servant. In private families, outside the sick room, it was hard to know what to do with her. She was neither for the kitchen nor for the drawing-room — neither fish, flesh nor fowl — and she was often placed in positions that required from her not only tact but a large amount of forbearance. But time has helped to settle the question and a trained nurse's position now is largely what she herself makes it. Occasionally, one still notices a trace of the old prejudice and of the feeling that a hospital nurse is not on an equality with other intelligent and refined women. Occasionally we still find families who consider it below their dignity that one of their members should enter a training school for nurses. Fortunately, however, this is largely a matter of education and I know by personal experience of many fathers and mothers, who, when once they had learned to appreciate the aims and duties of the trained nurse, were completely won over and encouraged their daughters when the latter wished to enter upon such a career.

Briefly, then, these are some of the stages through which the trained nurse has passed in the public estimation since she came into existence, until in these last days of the century, with its scientific medicine and modem hospitals, she is recognized as belonging to a profession, which has for its sphere the care of the sick, her work supplementing, not competing with, that of the scientific physician and surgeon.

But nurses are still reaching out towards ideals which we trust may be realized in the fullness of time. In speaking of nursing as a *profession* for women, I have used the term advisedly. Some prefer the term vocation, or the Anglo-Saxon word, calling. The last, if made to bear the significance of a direct call from God to a consecrated service, would rather suggest, on first thought, a sisterhood with its religious restrictions; and surely profession means all that vocation does and more. The work of the clergy, the lawyer and the physician is spoken of as a profession; the term implies more responsibility, more serious duty, a higher skill and an employment needing an education more thorough than that required in some other vocations of life. Every day these qualities are more and more being demanded of the trained nurse by modern physicians and by an exacting laity; and whether we recognize it or not, the fact remains that in so far as we fall short of meeting these requirements, in just such proportions are we found fault with and severely criticized.

Nor are the criticisms that we so often hear always unjust, for in glancing over the list of our attainments and summing them up there will be found room for much improvement. I think even the best among us are ready to acknowledge our imperfections, and the steady hard work that has been put into the past ten years in efforts towards improvements shows a healthy dissatisfaction and augurs well for the betterment of the future nurse. We cannot stand still; in the future the public, both medical men and the laity, will be ever demanding a still more efficient nursing, more uniformity, and a higher order of woman to meet these requirements. To be sure there are still to be found among the very conservative those who cannot become accustomed to the new order of things and who are not yet prepared to find the refined educated woman in the train id nurse; who do not comprehend the real difference between nursing as an occupation and as a profession. Their attitude would seem to be mainly due to the fact that they still labor under the impression that nursing consists chiefly in manual labor and that there is no necessity or scope afforded by it for a high degree of education. There are also those who proclaim that the old-fashioned nurse is good enough for them and maintain that nursing has not the first elements of a profession; they hold that the duties required of a nurse are very simple, that her education is complete when she has learned to make a bed and wash the patient, take the temperature and prepare the food, in fact to perform the ordinary duties for which any of the old-fashioned nurses were qualified. To distinguish between this popular idea of the care of the sick and to justify us in our pretensions to the rank of a profession we must consider the demands made by scientific medicine of today. Its methods are as different from those of the old-time practice as are those of modern nursing from the old-time nursing. Not so long ago neither medicine nor nursing were scientific in character. But the evolution of the one created a necessity for the other. Modern medicine requires a thorough scientific training and modern methods of treatment require that the work of the physician be supplemented by the constant and intelligent service supplied by the trained nurse, who has now her allotted part to perform in helping to carry cases of grave sickness to a successful termination. Thus, for example, it requires more than mere mechanical skill on the part of a nurse to follow the preparations for an aseptic operation, full of significance, as it is, in every detail, and the saying that "dust is danger" must have a bacteriologically practical meaning for her. At the present day, in all branches of surgery, the selection of a suitable operating-room nurse is no less important than that of any of the surgeon's staff. Nor can just anyone appreciate the full meaning of the physician when he says "the nursing will be half the battle in this case." Even the general public has come to recognize the important part that skilled nursing plays in such diseases as typhoid fever, pneumonia, and other forms of infectious disorders, because of the constant and intelligent care that must be given such patients.

To acquire not only the practical but also the theoretical groundwork of her profession, a woman must devote three of the best years of her life to special preparation and to obtaining a thorough understanding of the principles of nursing. Nothing can take the place of this training. It means all the difference that lies between the skilled, practiced worker and the amateur. Nursing has thus become a matter of scientific discipline and is a therapeutic agent of ever increasing importance. It is this education of the intelligence that constitutes the main difference between the trained nurse of today and the so-called nurse of former days, and that has rendered nursing worthy to rank as a department in scientific medicine.

To be sure there is the side to nursing so often spoken of as menial, but nothing dominated by the mind, and dignified by the way in which it is done, can be derogatory; nor need the cultured and trained woman, when the emergency arises, shrink from unpleasant tasks. The spirit in which she does her work makes all the difference. Invested as she should be with the dignity of her profession and the cloak of love for suffering humanity, she can ennoble anything her hand may be called upon to do, and for work done in this spirit there will ever come to her a recompense far outweighing that of silver and gold.

The trained nurse, then, is no longer to be regarded as a better trained, more useful, higher class servant, but as one who has knowledge and is worthy of respect, consideration and due recompense — in a certain degree a member of a profession. She is also essentially an instructor; part of her duties have to do with the prevention of disease and sickness, as well as the relief of suffering humanity. In district nursing we are confronted with conditions which require the highest order of work, but the actual nursing of the patient is one of the least of the duties which the nurse is called upon to perform for the class of people with whom she meets. To this branch of our work no more appropriate name can be given than "instructive nursing," for educational in the best sense of the word it should be.

These are some of the essentials in nursing by which it has come to be regarded as a profession, but there still remains much to be desired, much to work for, in order to add to its dignity and usefulness. As the standard of education and requirements become of a higher character and the training more efficient, the trained nurse will draw nearer to science and its demands and take a greater share as a social factor in solving the world's needs.

But there is another side to nursing — the ethical — without which all the work accomplished would be dead and spiritless, and which is the antidote for a too pronounced professional attitude. From this standpoint the nurse's work is a ministry; it should represent a consecrated service, performed in the spirit of Christ, who made himself of no account but went about doing good. The woman who fails to bring this spirit into her nursing misses the

pearl of greatest value that is to be found in it. Nor do such materialists in-
jure themselves alone, for they are the ones who bring upon our profession
the criticism, so often heard, that the life is apt to make a woman hard, cold
and mercenary. The scientific and educational side is important and should
certainly receive its due consideration, but none the less should each nurse
see to it that the spirit of love for the work's sake is fostered and developed,
in order that we may have a professional code of ethics of an eminently practical and helpful nature.

Such, then, are some of the responsibilities and privileges that each graduate assumes. A proper conception of our work carries with it the obligation
that each individual nurse, by her actions and by her personal character,
should do her part to maintain its dignity untarnished. To bring to it any less
than the very best that is in us will cause it to sink in the eyes of the public
and bring discredit both upon it and upon us. Nothing less than this individual high standard and interest will suffice, if we, as trained nurses, hope to
finally evolve an organization worthy in all respects to be ranked as a profession.

Chapter Three - Qualifications

When speaking of nursing as a profession, we discussed briefly the kind
and quality of the work to be done. In the natural order of things we now
pass on to the consideration of the kind of woman required to perform such
duties. In determining the standard of qualifications, many points have to be
carefully weighed, and while possibly some may think that unnecessary importance is attached to the preliminary requirements, it must be remembered that in the daily routine of a hospital, with its variety of patients, the
work of a nurse, even while herself receiving instruction, is not without its
immediate results. The hospital is her workshop, which she enters as a simple apprentice, it is true; but from the very first the preservation of human
life and the alleviation of human suffering are to some extent delivered into
her keeping. Can a woman, in any other kind of work which she may choose
for herself, find a higher ideal or a graver responsibility? Where human life
and health are concerned, what shall we term "the little things"?

Those of us who have had much experience in nursing, and know all we
would have a nurse to be, and how much she really must be, as the various
classes of women pass in review before our mental vision, will be inclined to
agree with the writer of a letter which came to me sometime since. After asking me to recommend a head-nurse for a hospital, and enumerating at length
the qualities she must possess to be successful, he concluded with the words,
"In short, we require an intelligent saint." A woman to become a trained
nurse, should have exceptional qualifications. She must be strong mentally,
morally, and physically; she must do thorough practical work; she must have

infinite tact, which is another name for a cultured common sense. She should be as one of the women of the Queen's Gardens in Ruskin's *Sesame and Lilies*, or such an one as Olive Schreiner describes, when she says, "A woman who does woman's work needs a many-sided, multiform culture; the heights and depths of human life must not be beyond her vision; she must have knowledge of men and things in many states, a wide catholicity of sympathy, the strength that springs from knowledge and the magnanimity that springs from strength." Only in so far as the women of our training schools attain to this standard will the institutions and communities, in which they labor, feel and show forth the influence of that "sweet ordering, arrangement and decision" that are woman's chief prerogatives.

Of mental endowments she can hardly have too many, but from a practical standpoint a good English education should be insisted upon. By this is meant that the candidate should come up to the standard required to pass the final examinations in the best high schools in the country, special stress being laid upon her ability to express herself, in writing or orally, with quickness and accuracy. Her knowledge of arithmetic should be of an eminently practical nature, so that she can readily deal with problems involving fractions, percentages, etc. This much is absolutely necessary. Of course more is always desirable, as no other study develops the reasoning powers in the same practical way, and women who know nothing in arithmetic beyond the few simple rules simply applied, are at once placed in a disadvantageous position upon entering upon their work in a modern hospital. Of course, if she has in addition a knowledge of bookkeeping, languages and a broad general reading, the candidate is all the better prepared for attaining to success in her career as a nurse.

Aside from this mental equipment, there are other qualifications of a practical nature that should be insisted upon. It would indeed be an advantage if every woman before entering upon hospital work could become a thoroughly trained housekeeper. Practical household economy should be a part of her home education, for in hospital wards the nurses are the stewards, the caretakers of the hospital property, and upon their thrift and careful ordering must depend the economical outlay of funds, which are really held in trust for poor and suffering humanity. I may be pardoned if I dwell more than once, and with what may appear to some to be too great an emphasis, upon the necessity of a knowledge of practical household economy. Experience has shown me to what a painful extent this branch of woman's work is neglected, or superficially understood, by so many women in all ranks of life. A total lack of, or appreciation for, the principles that govern such work will inevitably be followed by a deficiency in thoroughness and system. In the probationer evidences of this practical knowledge are readily recognizable; it will be apparent in the way she cares for her own room, her personal appearance, and in the order and system, which attend any work to which she puts her hand; moreover, her appreciation of the value of the articles with which, she has to work will be shown by the way in which she cares for them. Unfortunately, it too often happens that to training schools belongs the impossible task of teaching, in two or three short years, not only all that pertains to nursing, but also the first principles of domestic science. But when a graduate nurse goes into a private family and earns the just reproach of being extravagant and careless in the use of the property of others, and when the details of her work are without finish, the greater part of the blame should fall upon her early home training and not upon her school. That the importance to a nurse of a thorough knowledge of the principles and duties connected with housekeeping is becoming widely appreciated, especially by the authorities of training schools, upon whom unjustly falls the blame of her shortcomings in this respect, is evidenced by the fact that, in a few instances, superintendents in Europe and also in America have taken steps to provide a preliminary course of training for probationers, which embraces practical teaching in domestic economy, invalid cookery, anatomy and physiology, hygiene, and the elementary steps in nursing, before they are allowed to begin work in the wards of the hospital. This method commends itself as being so eminently practical and thorough, that it is to be hoped that all schools may adopt such courses at no distant a day. Again, as regards the probationer, this gradual introduction to her duties would go far to relieve her from any shyness and awkwardness, as well as dread, that she may have in first coming into contact with the sick. The principles of bed-making, bathing, cleanliness, disinfection, serving meals for invalids, the care of the lavatories, of the linen closet and its contents, of the kitchen and its various utensils, would all be familiar to her and she could at once proceed to put into practice, over and over again, these principles already learned, until she became expert in applying them. In this way not only would valuable time be saved to the probationer and to her head-nurse, but her thorough preparation for her duties would naturally conduce to the greater comfort of the patients, to the order and system of the ward, as well as helping all the other workers in it.

The selection of probationers is not a question of rank but of fitness; the college graduate who has never worked with her hands is just as undesirable in one sense as would be the applicant who has never had an opportunity for developing her mental powers, and has labored all her days with her hands — the one has what the other lacks, but both are one-sided. The woman, who would be a success as a nurse, needs the combined qualities of a trained mind and capable hands and body. Not until girls' schools and colleges supplement the home training, by offering to their students the opportunity of developing both hands and brain equally well, can we hope to meet every day with women who, so far as education can go, are fully equipped for entering a training school for nurses. But although progress sufficient to encourage us to persevere has already been made, the condition of affairs is by no means satisfactory. Rare, indeed, is the woman whose natural gifts and acquired qualifications entitle her to rank as an ideal candidate. Nor is it just that the defects in the nursing profession should be laid altogether at the door of the training schools. As things are now, these schools are too often called upon to make bricks without straw. They are expected to take average ability and cultivate it into something akin to the ideal. If the results are not always all one could desire, an honest inquiry would show that the difficulty lies very generally with the earlier education, the imperfections in which no hospital training can wholly eradicate.

I am aware that many think that nursing consists chiefly in manual labor and that there is no necessity or scope afforded by it for a high degree of education. Such persons, it would seem, fail to recognize that the opportunities for the trained nurse have increased and are growing every day. So wide a variety of important work is now offered to her and so much more is how required of her, that it would appear that she is restricted in her opportunities only by her own personal limitations. But even supposing that she keeps strictly to nursing as her life work, it is hardly possible for her to have too much education. As her knowledge grows, so will the interest in her work increase, because it can be done intelligently. Perhaps a few concrete instances will help to explain my meaning.

The development of bacteriology has done much to place medicine upon a scientific basis, and with it has arisen the necessity for a watchfulness over a variety of diseases, which requires a high order of intelligence and comprehension, the lack of which was, perhaps, not so important when drugs were considered cure-alls. The superficially educated woman with an untrained mind is at a distinct disadvantage in the wards of a modern hospital to-day. At present some of our remedial or preventive measures must appear to the uninitiated to be very vague and far-fetched, and since nurses after all are only human, the conscientious carrying out of them can hardly be expected, unless the intelligence is appealed to. What for instance are we to understand by cleanliness? For the uninitiated, the sense seems indeed to be very clear; and yet there is a deeper meaning, which can only be appreciated by those who have mastered at least the broad principles of bacteriology. How hopeless and dull, not to say irritating, would be the many washings and the various antiseptic applications, which are required from the nurse by the physician, unless she had learned from bacteriology to appreciate the fact that there exists a surgical, a microscopical, cleanliness. To fully appreciate the effect upon the patient of the air he breathes and the food he eats, she must know something of chemistry, ventilation and hygiene. For the proper care of the body she has to go to physiology; to become acquainted with the composition and the best forms and preparations of food, by which the greatest possible amount of bodily resistance to disease is established and maintained, she must supplement her knowledge of chemistry by the practical demonstrations of the diet school. Such matters of detail are usually entrusted to the nurse. She alone can devote to them such constant and unremitting attention as is necessary. It is true that the physician can lay down a broad general outline in such matters, but the details — the little things that matter so much — must of necessity be often left to the nurse; and how shall she supply all these without intelligence and a proper education in her profession; and how can she best utilize this special education, unless she brings to it a ground to build upon, a mind already trained to think and comprehend? I assert, then, that no woman can have too much preliminary education; even if she remains a private, as it were, in the ranks of the legion of trained nurses all her life, she need never fear that any part of her education will be thrown away.

The training school of a hospital may, therefore, be regarded as a place not only for fitting women to properly undertake the care of the sick, but as an educational institution, where properly selected women are given such moral and educational advantages that they can go forth equipped and ready to aid in the practical solution of some, of the various social problems, which are to be mastered only by the help of intelligent womanly work.

Health is another great essential, and though named last, is the first in importance; for no matter how acceptable a woman might be from the standpoint of education and personal goodness, these will avail nothing, if their possessor lacks the physical strength necessary for the work she assumes. Good health is a vital factor in the quality of the work performed, for the physical demands in caring for the sick are sometimes exceedingly arduous, and in the case of women who have not endurance, the strain of long hours and anxious watching cannot be sustained; and when the nurse's strength fails, the patient must suffer in proportion. All nurses need not be robust, but average health, at least, should be insisted upon, in the case of candidates. With this much as a foundation, provided that she always pays proper attention to the laws of personal health, a woman is more likely to be benefited than injured, in body as well as in mind, by following the prescribed hospital course.

The possession or lack of the ethical qualities, that belong to the make-up of the really good nurse, can only be discovered and those which are wanting be developed under the daily observation and criticism during the terms of probation and training.

To sum up her qualifications, *good physical health* is the first essential. The second is an *education,* which must not only be theoretical but practical; which, while comprising a knowledge of literature and science, should not have lacked the study of thrift and economy. But in addition to education she must have *culture.* This is, as a rule, a home product that has gradually been instilled into the young girl; without it she can possess only the shadow and not the substance. Kind and courteous to all, her demeanor must be characterized by a certain reserve. Her personal appearance is of importance; she need not be handsome or pretty; but in her dress, her hair, her adornment and her carriage, she should show her appreciation of what is fit and becoming. Her whole manner should suggest quiet, but at the same time a steady

22

firmness of purpose. She should be mentally, morally and physically well poised, "educated in the true sense of the word, so that what is most vital and admirable in her nature will have attained its legitimate development." Given these qualifications, I know of no occupation better adapted than nursing to render a woman self-reliant, of steady nerve, observant and responsible. The ranks of trained nurses should now and always be recruited from among healthy, cultured and properly educated women.

Chapter Four - The Probationer

The reasons that make women decide to enter a hospital to study to become nurses are probably as varied as the women themselves. Nor is the decision always based on a firm foundation, since it may have been arrived at as a result of a faulty knowledge of the subject. Hence it is highly desirable that a woman should be allowed to gain some insight into the life, which she believes she is fitted for, so that she can finally determine whether she will be doing right, or the reverse, in persevering in her determination. Hence the advantage to the candidate of the period of probation. It is probable that she may have read that a training in nursing is necessary, in order that she may be able to care for the sick and relieve suffering in the most skilful and humane way possible. But it often happens that she has not the remotest conception of all that is involved in such a training, and that a great many of her ideas are based upon mere theory. Close contact, however, with the work, even for a relatively short period, will convince her that, to become a good trained nurse, development must come from three sides — the hands, the heart, and the head. A few weeks will enable her to decide whether by long practice she can ever hope to be deft enough with her hands to do good work; whether her whole heart is in nursing, or whether she has been suffering from a temporary attack of emotion or sentimentality; and lastly, whether she can hope to obtain such a clear understanding of the fundamental reasons for all she does that, no matter how often she has to go over the same ground, she will be able to feel that she is condemned to no mere dull routine, but may always continue to grow, utilizing at every step and all the time developing, together with an ever-increasing manual dexterity, her intellectual and moral faculties.

On the other hand; from the Standpoint of the superintendent of the school, the amount of work a probationer could be made to accomplish is not of primary importance, the real object of the probationary period being to keep the would-be nurse and her work under daily observation a sufficient length of time to allow those, who are to be responsible for her future training, to judge whether the candidate possesses, in at least an average degree, the qualities that are necessary for the making of a good trained nurse; whether she is capable of learning what it will be necessary for her to know, and whether she is really in earnest in her desire to adopt nursing as a profession. In the majority of cases, these points can be settled in the course of a six weeks' or two months' probationary period by a superintendent who is practised in watching for the weak and strong points in character. At the same time, there are exceptions to this rule, and although one may have a distinct impression of what the general characteristics of a selected candidate are likely to be, one cannot always know what they really are, until she has been under observation for some months. Thus it sometimes happens that a probationer may be accepted, but dismissed, some months later, for the reason that she has at last shown the presence or absence of certain qualities which the test of experience and time alone could bring to light. In a certain sense, then, a woman always remains on probation during her whole term of pupillage and is subject to dismissal for cause at any time, although such extreme measures are adopted only when all others have failed to bring her up to the requirements.

The period of probation may be said to begin from the moment a probationer has been accepted and a definite date has been appointed for presenting herself at the hospital or training school. For whether she displays the quality of promptness by being businesslike enough to arrive on the day appointed, or fails to do so, will be reckoned for or against her in the final summing up. It is a matter of surprise how many women have not any appreciation of what is meant by punctuality. Unless for some exceedingly grave, unavoidable occurrence, a probationer should never fail to arrive on the day appointed, or ask to have the date changed. From the time her application is accepted, she becomes a unit in the training school, and although the work assigned to her in itself may be unimportant, any neglect or delay in keeping her compact cannot fail to cause inconvenience both to the superintendent and to others. Upon her arrival she will doubtless find someone ready to receive her and conduct her to the room she is to occupy for the time being. In the majority of schools she will very probably find that her room must be shared with another probationer or a recently accepted nurse. This arrangement has its advantages as well as disadvantages. For the newcomer the first few days in the school are usually somewhat dispiriting. She finds herself amid a number of other women, all of whom have their definite places and friends, and who seem so absorbed in what they are doing that they appear to be hardly aware that there is a stranger in their midst. Naturally, then, there is a certain fellow-feeling between new-comers and it is pleasant to find that there is some one else, who is equally a stranger to her surroundings. On the other hand, it may be a disadvantage to meet first with a new nurse, who has not yet learned discretion enough to prevent her giving a garbled description of hospital life, that may make the new arrival feel like taking herself and luggage off, without waiting to give her new career the test of personal experience.

In the nature of things a probationer must, of course, make mistakes. Everything is so new and strange, so different from any other position in life she has ever been in before, that the only wonder is she does not make more. But here, as at all other times, extremes must be avoided. The probationer must not allow herself to be too much cast down, nor on the other hand must she strive to get on too fast. The middle path will be found to be the safer, wiser, and in the end, easier; and the woman, who has sufficient intelligence and tact to take it, gives evidence at once of possessing adaptability and good sense. In the beginning it is better not to be familiar, over-eager to make acquaintances, too talkative, or too inquisitive. A moderate degree of silence and reserve befits the beginner. But the guarding of her tongue need not hinder her from observing quietly, but keenly, all that is going on about her, thus learning much to her advantage and at the same time showing that she is not deficient in the gift of quiet observation. If a probationer arrives early enough in the day, she should unpack her trunk, arrange her room and put on the dress she intends to wear in the ward. This should be of some washable material, neatly but plainly made, not too dainty, too much trimmed or too startling in color. In a word, her object should not be to attract attention, but in the arrangement of her hair, the neatness of her quiet dress and the absence of jewels of all kinds, she can show that she possesses a sense of the fitness of things and good taste.

According to the present arrangement in training schools, the probationer begins her duties in a hospital ward at once. She may, therefore, in the afternoon meet the head-nurse, under whom she is to work, be taken by her to the ward and introduced to the staff of nurses. The head-nurse will probably say a few words with reference to what the probationer is expected to do in beginning her regular work the next morning, may show her the lavatory and linen-room, and then assign her to some light duty, such as assisting in preparations for the patients' supper, or in opening beds for convalescents. At the nurses' supper hour the head-nurse, or some other nurse detailed to do so, will take the probationer back to the school, and see that she is shown to her place in the supper-room. Even here she is not free from observation, for if the superintendent takes her meals in the same room, she notices the table manners of each probationer; whether she reaches all over the table for what she wants, whether she drinks with her spoon in her cup, how she uses her knife and fork, — minor details, perhaps, when the grand work of nursing the sick is considered, but none the less signs of vast importance, since they show clearly what may be expected from a woman who, for some reason or other, has neglected to acquaint herself with the ordinary amenities of life. Sometimes, however, the probationer has not the good fortune to meet with this gradual introduction to her surroundings, but has to begin her duties in the morning. Then indeed she takes the plunge *in medias res*. She will find that her head-nurse will give her directions brief and to the point, if she does not turn her over entirely to the senior or some other assistant nurse. This beginning in the early morning hours is a harder test of her courage also, for she will not find the ward so attractive as later on in the day, when there is more evidence of leisure on every one's part, and when the rush and hurry of the morning's work and duties are over and the ward is quiet and presents its best appearance. Every hospital worker knows how much there is to be done after the night nurse goes off duty, and what a busy time it is in the wards until everything is all straight and in readiness for the regular visit of the medical staff. The importance of getting work done promptly will soon be impressed upon the new-comer; as soon as her share has been assigned to her, in order to get it done within the allotted time, she must learn to use despatch as well as thoroughness. But to do things quickly and thoroughly, method is all-important, and it will very soon appear whether a probationer possesses this gift in any degree. In a very few days her teachers will see whether the pupil begins to adopt methodical ways of setting about things, or whether she wastes a lot of time and labor in working vaguely in a disconnected way and is not adaptable enough to drop into the general routine of the ward work. Of course she must be allowed time to get over her first awkwardness and must not be too harshly criticized just at the start. Few of us will ever forget the feeling of utter Ignorance, helplessness and self-consciousness, that take possession of a new-comer in a ward, and how impossible and incomprehensible the medical terms and appliances are when one has first to do with them; moreover, the instinctive shrinking from the unpleasant sights, sounds and duties, and one's own helplessness and stupidity, seem to increase until one feels pretty well discouraged. Much, however, may be learned from quiet observation of the more advanced workers, and the happy, cheerful faces of the student nurses about her is encouragement enough for the right kind of a woman to persevere; they are sufficient evidence that her hour of discouragement will soon pass, if she is of the right metal to stand the test and go steadily on doing as well as she possibly can. Above all, let her remember to do what she is told to do, and no more; the sooner she learns this lesson, the easier her work will be for her, and the less likely will she be to fall under severe criticism. Implicit, unquestioning obedience is one of the first lessons a probationer must learn, for this is a quality that will be expected from her in her professional capacity for all future time. Some learn it with more or less difficulty; others never wholly master it; the happy few, who have been fortunate enough to have been trained to it from childhood, accept it naturally and never find it irksome. Thus, it not infrequently occurs that a head-nurse directs a probationer to leave the ward at a certain hour; the probationer, however, finding there is still much work to be done, probably out of mistaken kindness, or from a desire to help, takes it upon herself to remain beyond her time, until she is finally ordered off with a gentle reproof or the request to do only what she is told. I have also known probationers to be so impressed with the amount of work to be done in a ward that, instead of staying off duty for the specified time, they have returned an hour too soon, with the best intentions in the world of helping the work along by denying themselves the time for rest; unfortunately, when they have sometimes found themselves looked upon as officious and have been promptly requested never to return to the ward until the appointed hour, they have gone back with a feeling that they have been misunderstood and that their good intentions have not been appreciated. Now, in reality, they themselves only are to blame, inasmuch as they have failed to comply with two essential principles to be observed, if they are anxious for success, — implicit obedience and a habit of strictly minding one's own affairs. On the other hand, a probationer may be detained beyond her time when she thinks she ought to have been allowed to go off duty punctually; here again silence and quiet obedience are safest.

As a rule, it is the thoughtless, officious, interfering, opinionated woman, who is apt to fall under the displeasure of her head-nurse. The probationer may be unconscious that she possesses such undesirable qualities, never having been in a position before where she was obliged to restrain her tongue or the expression of her opinions; and when she meets with a rebuke, she is too apt to think that her head-nurse has taken a personal dislike to her; that other probationers in the ward are treated with more consideration; that more fault is found with her than with the others; that she is being sub-jected to a process of snubbing; she may even get the idea that the hardest and least attractive portions of the work are put off on her. As a result of this blindness to her own shortcomings, she feels bitterly hurt and may indulge in grumbling and gossip about her head-nurse with other probationers, in-stead of looking into herself for the cause of the trouble, where indeed it generally lies. It will be well for her to recognize the fact that this is the be-ginning of the discipline she must expect at the hands of one person or an-other more or less all through her professional life, and that it is under just such circumstances that the true interest and spirit in the work are manifest-ed. If a woman's sole object in becoming a nurse is the earning of so many dollars and cents; if she fails to bring with her any ideals as to the knowledge she may gain, or the ultimate good she may do, in becoming a nurse, to the shrewd observer this spirit will be made apparent by the manner in which the pupil accepts discipline. One would hardly think the commercial returns from the work of sufficient value to compensate for the constant and hard discipline a nurse must inevitably undergo.

The term of probation is calculated to discipline the beginner from the first, for the work she will be expected to do, at first sight, may appear to her unmitigated drudgery. Day after day she is drilled in the principles and vari-ous methods of making beds; day after day come the thorough dusting of everything in and about the ward, the care of lavatories and the various utensils, the cleansing of soiled rubber sheets, folding the ward linen and keeping the linen room in order, assisting in putting the ward in order after the physician's rounds, brushing up the wards or rooms at stated intervals, getting up and putting to bed convalescent patients, setting trays and serving meals, preparing patients for their meals, waiting upon them in minor ways, such as providing drinks or bed-vessels, and fetching and carrying in endless ways. Such work and services are almost never-ending in a ward of from twenty to thirty patients, and the probationer is required to do them over and over again, until she reaches a certain stage of thoroughness in regard to them and learns that each thing must be done not just any way, but that, there is a right way and that this is the one and the only one she must learn. The physical strain upon the probationer is at first very great. Unaccustomed to such constant hard work, towards the end of the day she is conscious of nothing but her weariness and aching feet; the bodily fatigue in its turn re-acts upon the nervous system, causing a feeling of depression, and she real-izes that hospital duties are very real, often very disagreeable and repugnant, with not a little drudgery about them. In all probability her preconceived ideas of her work have to be readjusted on a more practical basis and her enthusiasm must be tempered, although not quite quenched, before she fi-nally reaches a point where she begins to realize the necessity of learning thoroughly these foundation steps and appreciates the fact that she is gain-ing knowledge upon which to build the more responsible nursing work. And as the days go by and the end of the probation time draws near, she begins to find that all such things have their proper place in caring for the sick, and that nothing done for suffering humanity can be regarded as menial or mere drudgery, to be slurred over. Once having arrived at this point, instead of gladly availing herself of her privilege to leave at the end of the probation time, she eagerly and anxiously awaits the decision of the superintendent, whether she must go or whether she is allowed to stay. The tired feet and body are as nothing in comparison to the knowledge that she sees awaiting her, and to the conviction that this knowledge will give to her the right to join the ranks of those whose privilege it is to help to make the world better.

From the very start a woman begins to form habits in relation to her work which will be of ever-increasing value if they are good, but which, if bad, must inevitably be perpetual stumbling blocks. One of the ethical qualities a probationer should specially observe in connection with her work is *neat-ness*. From the very first bed made, from the very first article folded, she should make it the rule to strive to give a finished look to everything she does. In the matter of bed-making she should see that exquisite smoothness prevails, from the putting on of the first sheet to the tucking in of the ends of the coverlid and the adjustment of the pillows. Let this same neatness, order and system, be carried out by putting away at once in its proper place any-thing that has been used, in never allowing things to accumulate, in preserv-ing order at all times, in keeping a neat toilet-basket; in fact, she should make it a habit that everything, to which she puts her hand, should be left neat, clean, uniform and finished, for this means efficiency and accuracy in details in all branches of nursing work. The most trivial task, that has to do with the wellbeing of the patient, she must look upon as important and do it accord-ingly, giving it her best strength and thought, as well as her undivided attention, so that it may be done in the very best known way. This does not necessarily mean that a great deal of time should be expended; on the contrary, another habit most important to acquire is to be dextrous with one's hands, with a quiet, gentle swiftness which should be the outcome of repeated, untiring efforts. Let her be faithful in the very least things and the graver, greater things will be sure to be taken care of.

Punctuality has already been mentioned and will be again referred to later. Talking too freely over one's ward experiences with other probationers, and faultfinding about things one cannot possibly understand all the reasons for in so short a time, should be avoided. Lastly, a proper regard for the *hospital etiquette* will be required of her. For the probationer this will chiefly consist in being courteous to all with whom she comes in contact in an official way, in the hospital and training school proper, being careful not to make in any direction any unnecessary advances. Towards the patients, with whom she will have less to do than later on when she becomes a pupil, she should deport herself as she proposes to continue,, with due consideration in all respects, remembering they are the first reason for her being in the hospital and should, therefore, always receive her first consideration and care. Towards fellow probationers and the other nurses in the ward it is best not to be too familiar, or too friendly; sudden, violent friendships are undesirable and unnecessary. Later on, when she has been accepted as a pupil, she will have time enough to form friendships; until then the ordinary courtesies are all that are necessary. In the wards, if obliged to come in contact with the patients' friends or with strangers, the probationer should always refer them to the head-nurse or whoever may be in charge of the ward. She should never assume unnecessary responsibility. With the physicians a probationer will have but little to do and all that is required at her hands is to carry out orders. Any attention coming from the students or members of the medical staff, who may be working in or about the ward, should not be encouraged, for every woman who enters a hospital must remember that henceforth she walks in the gaze of the public, subject to the observation and criticism of all classes of people and that she must deport herself accordingly. The ordinary little attentions and social privileges, that she may have been accustomed to in the small social circle at home, cannot be permitted in the large wards of a hospital. She is there for other and grave reasons; and for her own sake and for the sakes of her fellow-workers she must strive to walk worthy of her vocation in all respects. The rules of the institution should be strictly observed; not that at first she will understand them all, but she may be sure there is a good reason for most of them; moreover, to observe them should be a point of honor with herself, and it is certain that the lesson in discipline and obedience she may learn from simply keeping the rules may be of the greatest value to her. Talking while on duty, is not allowed for the reason that there is not time for it, nor is the ward the place to indulge in any topics not bearing directly upon the work on hand, which needs one's undivided attention and thoughts.

A probationer will find that a certain military precision exists in regard to the deportment of a junior to those who are her superiors in office. Thus it is considered only courteous to stand when receiving an order or upon being spoken to by the superintendent, the head-nurse, or a physician; but to feel obliged to stand all the time a doctor is in the ward is not necessary. A probationer may go on quietly with her work, whether she be standing or sitting, unless she is being directly addressed. Unnecessary questions, talking and noise, are strictly prohibited during the rounds of the medical staff, since such interruptions are not courteous and may interfere with their observations on the patients. A probationer has always the privilege of asking her head-nurse questions regarding her work, but she should use judgment in selecting her times for so doing. Upon coming on duty she should always report at once to the head-nurse, or whoever is in charge of the ward, and again when the hour arrives for leaving the ward.

A two months' drill in hospital work and etiquette, if properly utilized, cannot fail to leave any woman with a broader and more practical outlook upon life, and is a very necessary test and preparation for any one who would take upon herself the graver responsibilities and duties of a pupil-nurse.

Chapter Five - The Junior Nurse

With the donning of the uniform the probationer completes the first stage of her hospital training and is transformed into the pupil-nurse, whose instruction will extend over a period not merely of weeks but usually of three years. During the first year of her training she is known as a junior nurse, and is one of the junior class, whose members have their own distinct place and duties in the work of the hospital. They have their own courses of lectures, classwork, demonstrations and examinations, and the class begins at once to make its own traditions, better or worse than those of the class preceding it — traditions which are likely to be remembered and handed down for the edification or admonition of generations of classes not yet formed. Each new pupil-nurse becomes at once identified with her own class, and it is the wisest plan for her to find her interests in it from the first, to look for her intimate friends there, and to do her full share in working for good traditions. It is a mistake to seek friendships wholly beyond one's own circle. A nurse who has to go outside of her own class for friends and social intercourse, or who consorts too freely with the new probationer, shows that she is lacking in some of the qualities that make people attractive and desirable as friends; moreover she is apt to be regarded with suspicion by those in authority, and in the end such conduct will tell against her. There is a vast difference between showing a probationer kindness and due consideration and in being on terms of intimacy with her. Besides, it is not good for the probationer to be admitted into too close an intimacy, until she has proved herself worthy of entire confidence.

The junior nurse is first instructed in the principles of nursing by means of systematic classes, lectures and demonstrations; but it is in the wards that she has an opportunity to daily and hourly put these methods and principles into practice, until she makes them entirely her own. A junior nurse must ever bear in mind that, from her standpoint, the main object of the work she is required to perform in a ward is not so much for the sake of getting a certain quantum done no matter how, as that she may have an opportunity of doing the same things over and over again, until they could not possibly be done better by anyone else. Thus, each time she has a piece of work to do, she should always remember to try and do it just a little better, more quickly and more deftly than she did it the last time. She should make a bed, tidy up a ward, give a bath, comb a patient's long hair, make a poultice, do everything in fact always on this principle of doing it better; each time should be regarded as an opportunity, and the oftener the better; and though she may sometimes grow physically tired, that is a secondary matter. A pupil should esteem it a piece of good fortune to be put on duty in the heavy wards, where one is always busy, where the work never seems to be done, and where there is so much in the way of nursing going on. She should look upon the assignment as a splendid opportunity, instead of feeling downcast or grumbling over it. Never be afraid to work and to work hard. Work pure and simple is not likely to do you harm; as a rule, mind and body feel the strain only when one tries to combine it with too many other interests. Never seek for the soft spots or the easy places in hospital work; if you get them, you will surely lose golden experiences that will be regretted bye and bye, when the opportunity is gone beyond recall. Only by constant repetition can you become really familiar with the work; only by doing a thing well again and again can you obtain confidence, accuracy and precision. It is this constant, intelligent practice that constitutes the difference between the skilled, trained, professional woman and the amateur. Despite the common use of the term, the "born nurse" does not exist; no amount of theory by itself will avail; it will always be necessary to take hold of each task and do it over and over again, being guided and dominated by an intelligent, trained mind and a willing spirit. It is true that one woman may have a greater natural liking for nursing and more aptitude for study than another and so learns more quickly and better; but no one, however gifted, can have too much practical experience in the art of caring for sick people.

During the first year the pupil has many opportunities allowed her of a practical nature, for she is expected to become expert in bed-making of all kinds, in giving all the various baths, in caring for a bed-patient in every detail, in administering medicines and foods, in making the various external applications, in the use of appliances, and in bandaging, besides learning the principles of invalid dietary. She also assists at the medical staff's visits, and gets a thorough drill in the details of such rounds from her head-nurse, during which she learns something of the nature of disease and its treatment. She becomes impressed with the necessity for method, order and forethought, as well as a knowledge of all the details about so many patients; as a consequence, she learns to be careful, watchful and observant and to keep her head-nurse informed about everything concerning the patients assigned to her; she recognizes the fact that every detail may be of great importance and acts accordingly. She also learns to be thoughtful for the patients in many little ways that at first do not occur to her, but only come as she by degrees forms the habit of watching for opportunities to add little comforts to the usual routine of what is done for them. She gradually realizes that all such little attentions are in a way medicines, which go far towards hastening a patient's recovery; that the prescribing and administering of these rest with herself and that much depends, therefore, upon the amount of interest she takes in her patients. So busy and absorbed does she become in her duties and surroundings, that she loses sight of self, which becomes of secondary consideration in comparison with her work, until she suddenly realizes that four whole months of her year have gone and she is brought face to face with her first great responsibility in being assigned to her first night-duty.

But before discussing this important service, we will consider another form of education that should go hand in hand from the very beginning with the practical training and teaching, and that must be attended to just as diligently as any part of her technique, if the pupil hopes to finally become an all-round nurse of a high order, whose perceptive faculties are so finely trained as to know by intuition, as it were, what conduces to her patient's comfort.

The cultivation of certain habits of body and mind should be begun with the first putting on of her uniform, for the acquisition of a habit of any kind necessitates time and persistent effort. The systematic study of the subjects dealing with the ethical side of nursing work should be regarded as most important, until the principles involved have become the mainspring which controls her every action. There are many desirable attributes that a woman may have from the beginning — the more the better — and many others that she will insensibly acquire from the very nature of her work, her surroundings and the school traditions. But as she gradually learns what is necessary, she should make sure that she is ever trying to develop more highly those qualities, which she already possesses, and to acquire those in which she feels herself lacking.

A nurse's *personality* is a factor that can never be disregarded, owing to its influence upon the patient. Moreover, the possession of the attributes that make up our personality — rendering it pleasant or the reverse — depends largely upon ourselves. Certain qualities of mind and body may be born in us, but it is always in our power to modify or increase their significance. For all of us it is desirable to improve our natural gifts, but in the case of a nurse it is absolutely necessary that she should have under her control such character-istics of body and mind as may affect or influence for good or bad her pa-tient's condition. This is particularly true in reference to the expression of the face, the quality of the voice, the character of the touch or footstep, and to the carriage of the body in general. There is always a spiritual or mental de-velopment or change taking place within us, that is shown to the outside world through the medium of the body, the inward workings of the mind be-ing rendered visible through the various motions consciously or uncon-sciously employed. It is difficult to realize at first how susceptible a patient is to the various expressions which may appear in the faces of the physician and nurse; how closely he watches their every action, in the hope that he may gain a clue as to what they really think of his condition, and how much he is encouraged or cast down by what he thinks he reads there. Hence it is all important, from the very outset, to study to keep well in hand one's vari-ous modes of expression and to watch them with unceasing diligence, until the habit of self-control becomes second nature and the chances of being caught off one's guard are reduced to a minimum.

The face, eye, voice, touch and movements should all receive attention, for it would avail but little if one learned to control the expression of the face, or the glance of the eye, only to be betrayed by the tone of the voice, a shrug of the shoulders, a disagreeable touch or by the general deportment. Nor will there be lacking opportunities of judging what progress is being made in this respect, for only a nurse of long experience knows what profound self-control is sometimes required to keep one's true feelings from coming to the surface. To always yield a cheerful and prompt obedience to those in authori-ty and to gave up one's own will; to learn to adapt one's self to a community life; to keep up pleasant relations with other nurses, some of whom may be uncongenial, but with all of whom she has to work in harmony; to render a ready compliance to the many little and seemingly capricious demands of patients — especially when they come at the end of a long day's work, when her own back is aching and her feet are tired or when she may not be feeling well herself — all these must be looked upon as affording opportunities for self-control and self-discipline. The true nurse must be "all things to all men." To-day her duty may require her to be the sustaining presence at a grave cri-sis or at a death-bed; to-morrow she is called upon to share in the rejoicings over the newborn child, or to encourage and cheer the convalescent. To be bright and to look cheerful and happy can hardly be regarded as of great merit in a woman when she is feeling fresh and strong, but it is a victory if she can appear so when she is feeling just the reverse, and when it requires no little exertion to maintain a cheerful atmosphere.

The *face* should be trained never to show a trace of anxiety or alarm, no matter how grave the occasion; no surprise should be expressed even by so much as the lifting of an eyebrow, no dissatisfaction or displeasure. Tranquil and impassive, — which does not, however, mean having a stony expression — the face should never tell tales, whereby harm may result to the patient, but should habitually express cheerfulness, kindliness and quiet solicitude. Smiles are not hard to cultivate, and like mercy stand in good stead to the giver and receiver —to nurse and patient. But even smiles may be overdone and fall flat when they are meaningless and artificial, or when they are of the spasmodic, nervous kind that partake of the nature of a grin.

A well trained *eye* adds greatly to the powers of observation. This point is dwelt upon at length in textbooks on practical nursing, in so far as it concerns symptoms belonging to the various diseases. But here should be emphasized the importance of training the eye to be on the alert, so that it observes everything that may add to the patient's comfort or pleasure, be it ever so little. But while the nurse should be quick to discern any change in the patient's condition, no matter how startling this may be, the eye should keep its secret. To the patient it should ever appear calm, steady, clear, vigilant, an eye that conveys confidence, and a sense of security, a feeling that someone is watching his interests all the time.

Nor is the quality of the *voice* an unimportant matter, although there seems to be an impression abroad that this is the one organ over which one can have no shadow of control, unless it be to reduce it to a whisper. Thus we meet with nurses who either speak through their noses, or deep down in their throats in guttural tones; others have an indistinct utterance; they mumble, are hard to understand and the tone of the voice is deficient in firmness. The harsh, loud, discordant voice, which would grate even upon well ears, and the quick, sharp, imperative tone, or the high, shrill piercing variety, are all too common. Again, some women talk, as it were, in nervous jerks; they repeat their words or stammer over their sentences; while others are characterized by an apathetic drawl or its opposite, the hard metallic voice — both conveying a lack of sympathy, interest and innate kindliness of nature. Lastly, there is the plaintive, sad, subdued tone that sounds as though its owner is always on the point of weeping. Any of these defects are quickly noted by the sick; they jar upon nerves that are unstrung, sick and out of tune themselves. Fortunate, indeed, is the woman who, in starting out in her career, possesses a well-modulated voice. But as regards those who have not been gifted by nature in this respect, I would insist that up to a certain point the defect is unpardonable, since it is perfectly possible to cultivate a quality of voice that at least will not be offensive, while by thought and practice a fair degree of sweetness can be attained. Thus, when we meet with a nurse who possesses a disagreeable quality of voice, we are perfectly justified in ascribing the defect to ignorance, indifference or carelessness. For the sick-room we need a voice that is uniformly even, quiet, low but distinct, sweet but firm, with a cheery strain in it, that encourages and makes the patient feel better in spite of himself. A well-modulated voice is a power in itself, "to sooth, to comfort and command." The quiet note of authority is necessary, for it conveys a sense of strength and helpfulness that reacts favorably upon patients and to which they readily yield. Sick people are like children in some respects; they quickly recognize a stronger power than themselves and obey it with better grace. But they are also like children in their desire for sympathy and are keen to discover its absence or presence, through the expression of the face, but more particularly through the voice. The popular idea still prevails widely that, when anyone is ill, he should be whispered to, or whispered over, in an awesome, mysterious tone of voice. It is strange that people never seem to find out that sick people resent such treatment; their suspicions are readily aroused; to them the whispering means that they are worse or very ill indeed; they want to know all that is being said about themselves. Never say in a sick person's presence what you do not want him to hear; and never whisper over him; speak distinctly but quietly, and stand near enough to the bed to be both seen and heard. On the other hand, I have seen patients treated as though sudden deafness had seized them with the illness, the friends and attendants literally shouting at them in tones which would have awakened the seven sleepers.

It is not always an easy matter to control the tone of the voice when one is displeased or tired, or has been very much tried by patients or their friends. Sometimes it requires a distinct effort to keep the harsh, discordant note from becoming apparent. But it is worth while to control oneself, for the next time the task will not seem so hard. When one is feeling out of sorts, it is always well to keep silent as much as possible, although never to the point of appearing sullen. One has to be very guarded in one's conversation, and learn the value of both silence and speech. It is not necessary to entertain a patient all the time by talking to her. But although the desire to talk incessantly, or to make unnecessary comments, should always be controlled, on the other hand, it is always polite to show either by speech or sign that one has been spoken to. It is exasperating to the well, and much more to the sick, to have a remark or a suggestion treated with sullen silence or indifference. Such behavior represents a form of rudeness that is intolerable.

A junior nurse may begin to practice this habit of discreet silence by restraining her desire to talk at meals, or in her room at night, over the various experiences she has met with during the day. In fact one great evil, which exists in our training schools, consists in the tendency to talk over hospital experiences at table, and to spend leisure time, which could be much better employed, in congregating in one another's rooms and further embellishing such tales, or in dwelling upon the doings and short-comings of head-nurses, fellow-nurses, the superintendent, or members of the medical staff. This pernicious habit cannot be too severely censured, for the reason that after two or three years of such indulgence the woman is left with an appetite for gossip; she becomes indiscreet and unsafe to be trusted with either institution or family affairs. When a nurse recognizes a disposition on the part of the members of her class to indulge in such conversation, her best plan is to quietly withdraw for the time being. Better to be alone and silent than to run the risk of acquiring such a disagreeable habit.

In the sick room the nurse's speech should be controlled by a sense of the fitness of things. She should be very circumspect in her own language, and encourage nothing from patients, or their friends, that borders on familiarity, vulgarity, or frivolity. Wit and humor should be kept well in hand and should be of the kind that never hurts. Slangy expressions or unseemly jests should not be indulged in. Even with one's fellow nurses too much familiarity should not be allowed in the way of teasing, practical jokes, and the like. Such things are "not convenient," nor are they in keeping with the character of a nurse and nursing work. Be constantly refined in all manner of conversation; never allow familiarity with disease to betray you into making or countenancing so-called professional jokes. It is indeed sad that death itself is sometimes made the subject of a gruesome jest. Avoid using abbreviations for medical terms, where the whole word should be used. Thus, hypo., mag. sulph., strych. sulph., D. & C, and the like, sound slangy, slip-shod, undignified, and the style smacks of illiteracy.

No less than the voice should the *sense of touch* be rendered a carefully cultivated adjunct to one's work. One cannot very well change the size or shape of the hand, but one can largely control its touch. Sick people are as acutely sensitive in regard to the character of the touch as they are to the quality of voice, and respond to it just in proportion as it conveys to them a sense of skill and gentleness, sympathy and carefulness. Moreover, the presence of these qualities goes far towards reconciling a troublesome patient to the various necessary manipulations. The importance of training the hands to do things deftly, swiftly and with accuracy, can hardly be over-estimated; from the patient's standpoint, there is all the difference in the world between having things done by one who possesses this deftness and skill and by one who works haphazard. In the former case everything goes on smoothly with no unnecessary loss of time or undue haste. Thus, for example, in giving a bath, every portion of the body is gone over with the same smooth firm motion; the skin is well dried; the hair is combed without pulls and snarls; the bed is made without repeated turnings, pullings and twistings; the room is tidied up without noise and apparently arranges itself, so that, when all is done, there remains a sense of comfort, rest and quiet. On the other hand, the bath is given in patches, and when it is finished, the patient feels as though some spots had never been touched, while others were only half dried; added to this, all the manipulations have been gone about so slowly and in such a clumsy way that the water, which possibly at first was too hot, has finally cooled too much; the hair is brushed in a jerky, fitful way; snarls are tugged at not too gently, so that at the end the patient is left with a headache. The bed-making, too, is a source of discomfort and the tidying-up of the room sets the nerves on edge. The process is so long and tedious; various articles are constantly being dropped; the bed is jarred every time the nurse passes it. As a result of these annoyances, the patient is too nervous and tired to settle down for her nap and she is left with a sense or irritation that may not wear off for the entire day.

A sensitiveness of touch should be acquired so that one may have one more aid in perceiving quickly, even in the dark, any material change in the bodily condition of the patient. It should at all times be gentle, showing sympathy and tenderness, soft and magnetic in its power to sooth the nervous restless patient or to lull her to sleep.

In the same way one's *hearing* should be trained to be keen to note every sound that comes from the sickbed. Frequently it happens that, when the ear can catch the regular breathing of the patient, the nurse feels reassured and knows that all is going on well. When the lights are turned low, it would annoy the patient to turn them up frequently in order to make our observations.

The character of the *walk* should always be considered, as this also is within our power to control. A light, even, firm, elastic tread does not depend upon the stature, but upon decision of mind. Some women have by nature a slow, indolent, dragging walk, with which their work is usually in keeping; others have a heavy, loud, vigorous, commanding foot-step, of whose disagreeable qualities the owner seems quite unconscious. Then there is the nurse who is on the half-run all the time, but accomplishes very little; another has a funny little trotting gait, hesitating, broken and uncertain; she is always anxious to do well, but falls short in her efforts; or again, we have the quick, nervous, sharp step, and the mincing, tip-toe walk. All of these and many more come to my mind as I write; and the impression made by them on the patients is very vivid and lasting. Tip-toeing is particularly objectionable, as it emphasizes the fact of illness and is consequently bad in its effect upon the patient. The foot-fall of a nurse may be soothing or it may have quite the contrary effect. The everyday, quiet, even, straight ahead gait is perhaps the best to aim at and is the least noticeable, if it can be attained.

It is through the exercise of a happy combination of all these powers that the general actions are regulated. Through them we can also convey a *sympathy* of the wise, helpful, unobtrusive kind, which is shown not so much in words as by the expression of the face and eye, the touch of the hand, the tone of the voice, the unfailing gentle speech, and the atmosphere of interest, care and thoughtfulness, which the true nurse takes with her into the sick room and which characterizes her every action. The usually unobservant person is keenly alive to the absence or presence of sympathy in those who nurse him. He is swift to distinguish whether he is being treated as a, more or less interesting case or as an individual; whether he is of first or secondary importance in the nurse's thoughts and feelings. But sympathy and tenderness are never synonymous with familiarity of manner. It is quite possible for a nurse to be gentle and sympathetic with her patients, without being familiar.

Again, as influencing and emphasizing the actions, *manners* must be considered. The nature of her work, the character of her surroundings, as well as her position, require the careful observance on the part of a nurse of a professional attitude. Her demeanor should be characterized by an unfailing courtesy to all, familiarity with none, and a dignity and reserve that should be hers by virtue of her office as a nurse; in a word she must possess good breeding, which is mainly a home product, to be cultivated from earliest childhood. One possessed of this essential instinctively fits her behavior to the occasion and readily understands the necessity for drawing the line between professional and social manners in her work and of not confusing courtesy with familiarity. This distinction should be more felt than seen, and there should always be present that little invisible barrier of dignity and self-respect, that in its turn commands respect from others. This real dignity, while not permitting rudeness to or from another, does not insist upon the recognition of a fancied importance, nor does it assume an air of superiority, but on the contrary is natural, quiet and unpretending.

A good professional manner should be maintained in the hospital ward at all times. A nurse should treat her equals with courtesy, those superior to her m official rank and authority with deference, and accord to them a willing obedience. From the head-nurse down, every member of the nursing staff, while on duty, should regard herself as the assistant of the medical staff in the care of the sick and should be punctilious never to overstep these official restrictions nor permit visits and conversation in the ward not connected with her duties. It must be remembered that the relations of nurse and doctor are purely professional and that a hospital ward is the last place for social intercourse or attentions, which must inevitably lower the professional dignity of the entire nursing staff. A woman of good common sense and refinement will understand the discipline and etiquette that are enforced in all good schools in this respect, and will cheerfully observe any rules, written or unwritten, in regard to it.

Toward strangers, who may be present in a ward for any reason, a nurse should show the utmost courtesy and make them feel welcome, no matter how busy or pressed for time she may be. With a junior nurse this courtesy need by no means take the form of making statements about the ward or patients; she must be discreet in volunteering information, and should refer her questioners to the head-nurse. Good sick-room manners, — everything we do that relates directly or indirectly to the patient — are the outcome of forethought, consideration and self-control, which result in a certain graciousness not otherwise present. A nurse is in the sick-room for a definite purpose; she should, therefore, bring all her skill to bear in order to succeed in that purpose, and for this more than merely technical nursing is required of her. She may undo all the good her technical skill should do, by her manner of doing her work. It is all-important to gain the goodwill and confidence of her patients, and in this connection manners stand for much. To be companionable a nurse must have a bright disposition, a serene, quiet cheerfulness, coupled with gentleness and decision of manner. Loudness and noise should be avoided, a harsh and abrupt, or a hurried, fussy, excited manner grates upon the nerves. One should study to be quiet, deft and quick. Sick people generally are very easily disturbed by noise, and the sense of hearing is sometimes abnormally acute in illness, so that even ordinary sounds may cause positive suffering. Doors should be opened and closed with an almost reverent touch — swiftly but noiselessly; they should never be left unfastened, so that they are liable to continuously creak or bang. In fact all the machinery of the sick-room should be well oiled, as it were, and should be regulated with carefulness and a quiet, intelligent routine, which does not admit of noise and which does not worry or excite the patient. It would be impossible to enumerate the many ways in which a nurse may be noisy, although memories of shortcomings in this respect would fill pages. More particularly, however, the fact might be emphasized that, when off duty, nurses in general seem to think it is their privilege to throw off all restraint and to become even more than ordinarily noisy, showing an utter disregard for the comfort of others, especially of the night-nurses, who may be trying to sleep on the same floor. A nurse should at all times guard against such behavior. The restriction is one of the sacrifices, if she so regards it, which she must willingly consent to when she chooses her profession.

A nurse should carry herself with an almost military air of erectness and alertness — the evidences of a well-disciplined body. Too many have a habit of lounging and loitering about as though they were deficient in back-bone, like jelly-fish. They seem to be looking almost instinctively for something to support them. They usually lean against the patient's bed, when talking to the occupant, or when the doctor is making his visit, if they do not actually sit down. Their whole demeanor indicates inertia, except that they are probably diligent users of the rocking-chair in the patient's room. On the other hand, we have the other extreme. Some women want to be too quick; they are clumsy, and in their haste are forever running into things; they can never go near the patient's bed without knocking against it; they cannot pick up anything without dropping it again; these are all evidences of lack of discipline or pure carelessness. Peculiar mannerisms must be overcome; a little mincing way of doing things and a stiff uncompromising attitude are equally objectionable.

In the matter of table manners one cannot be too careful not to allow one's self to grow careless of the little attentions, courtesies and niceties which belong to civilized society. For this reason, before entering the dining room, the nurse should always be careful to remove her apron and sleeves, in which she has been doing all manner of work about the sick, or to change her operating-room dress for the regular uniform. The habit of reaching over the table for what is wanted should be avoided, as well as loud laughing, talking and too much haste. Amid the hurry and demands of institution life there is always a temptation to be careless in trifles; but this tendency should not be yielded to, for in time the giving way to it leads to the formation of objectionable habits. It ought not to be said of any nurse that she fails to give satisfaction, whether from ignorance or carelessness, in her social manners.

I have taken pains to dwell at some length upon these primary ethical points which a nurse should possess, because just in proportion to their presence or absence will be the measure of true success. But the method of acquiring good habits is quite a different matter and rests almost entirely with the woman herself. It is impossible to lay down any one rule dealing with the development of all these ethical principles. Careful training, congenial surroundings, good traditions will do much, but the results will always be mediocre, unless the woman brings into her training the *true spirit of nursing*, upon which to build her education and experience. We form our estimate of her character from her deeds, but these are only the outward expression of the measure of the inward spirit of love for her work and for humanity. If her main purpose is based on high ideals, the development of sterling ethical attributes will be the direct fruit, and true devotion to her duties and her responsibilities will never be lost sight of. Selfishness will have no part in her life. The various other selfs, too, will find their proper places — self-control, self-reliance, self-possession — while self-abnegation, though ever present, will be lost sight of entirely by one who has learned to regard her duties not as sacrifices but as pleasures and privileges, to be met in a spirit of cheerfulness, willingness and love. And through this spirit of willingness and devotion will come the proper kind of discipline — the discipline of self — which will render that demanded by the hospital the more readily understood, appreciated and accepted, and will result in the right preparation for the more varied and exacting discipline of the outside world.

The reading about such requirements may have a hard sound and their attainment may at first seem impossible, but the actual accomplishing comes about in a gradual, almost unconscious fulfillment. The path is long and thorny, but to those who tread it aright the final outcome will be a strong, attractive personality, faculties well in hand, a temper well under control, a high degree of toleration towards others, an even, cheery, gentle disposition, a refined, gracious manner and a devotion to duty.

Such a personality — equally good all through — is not only inspiring and helpful to the patient, but stimulates all who come in contact with it. I have in mind nurses, who have been great successes because of their cheerful, hopeful dispositions and ready adaptability, although their practical nursing was far from the highest order. Such instances in themselves would teach that a due regard for ethical responsibilities is just as important as practical proficiency, for there are no circumstances, in which a woman is placed, where her individuality stands out more sharply, or where her personal influence is more felt than in the sick-room. Such qualities should be cultivated and developed in the course of hospital training with courage, endurance and perseverance, "until labor and duty lose all the harshness of effort; until they become the impulse and habit of life when, as the essential attributes of the beautiful, they are, like duty, enjoyed as a pleasure."

Chapter Six - Health - The General Care of the Body

A discussion on personality would be incomplete without a reference to the vital part played in it by the physical condition. A woman, who has been accepted as a pupil in a training school, presumably begins her work with average health; if she exercises proper care during her training, she will find herself at the end of her time better and stronger physically than when she began. This result is mainly due to the regular life she leads, to the regular exercise she gets in the performance of her routine duties, to the constant occupation of the mind and body, and to the sound sleep at night which naturally follows, to a careful observance of the laws of health, and to a certain freedom from, or at least a division of, responsibility. It would be of vital importance that a nurse should pay particular attention to the care of her health, if only for the reason that the loss of it would hamper her in carrying on her profession. To try and do nursing work without at least fair health would be an act of folly; without health her work must cease and the order of things is reversed; she becomes the patient instead of the nurse. Unless she has a sound mind in a sound body, she cannot care for her patients properly; even slightly impaired health will render the quality of her work inferior. From another point of view it is also her distinct duty to keep herself well. In a hospital nurses are provided in proportion to the work to be done; when one is taken ill, her share of the work has naturally to be assumed by the others, who thus have extra duties to perform. Again, if a nurse is only half well, she does her work superficially, and either the patient suffers or the burden falls upon other shoulders. Furthermore, inasmuch as bad physical health always involves an inferior mental condition, she will be in no state to exercise good judgment or to assume responsibility. The spirit may be willing enough, but when the flesh is weak and feeble, the results cannot be good. Nor is it just that patients should be cared for by a half-sick person, for if they are not altogether heartless, they may harm themselves in trying to save the nurse, and may even refrain from asking for the necessary care, lest they should overtax her powers. Of course this is not right, and the proper authorities should always see that patients are protected from this form of imposition. In order to do her duty by her patient, then, the nurse must understand and observe the proper care of herself. That she is never wanting in this respect is usually assumed by outsiders and the public generally. Superintendents of training schools are, perhaps, the only ones who could testify to the contrary and who know what a difficult task it is to bring nurses to a sense of their duty as regards giving proper attention to their health. In hospitals, in particular, it is the exceptional case, when a nurse becomes ill, that her sickness cannot be traced back to some act of indiscretion on her own part, to the disregard of the rules laid down to suit her special needs, to some wilful act of carelessness, or to the formation of habits contrary to the laws of health.

Some people seem to have a peculiar gift for forgetting what is told them or not obeying orders to the letter. For instance, one of the minor physical troubles a woman may develop, when she first enters a training school, is a sore throat — the so-called hospital sore-throat — which, if neglected, may result in an attack of tonsillitis, which takes her off duty and confines her to bed for at least three or four days. Such an attack can in almost every instance be averted, if the nurse obeys her superintendent and tells her on the first day she finds her throat even slightly sore. Unfortunately, it usually takes more than frequent tellings — an attack of tonsillitis — before this fact can be impressed on the nurse's mind, and she often comes to report only on the second or third day, and when she can hold out no longer. Her excuse for not saying anything about the matter sooner is usually that she did not wish to give trouble. But she has not taken into account the fact that her absence from duty for three or four days, or even a week, is in the end infinitely more inconvenient for everybody concerned. Again, a really serious illness means endless trouble in many directions, a special nurse, sometimes two, so that there will be two or three nurses less to care for the patients, not to mention untold extra work and planning for the superintendent. Now, of course, it is not meant that a nurse can always keep well, and provided that an illness follows as the direct result of devotion to duty, no treatment can be too good for her, and all that physicians and fellow-nurses can do for her is only her right. Just now I am referring to avoidable sickness. When a nurse falls ill in a hospital, she usually commands an undue amount of sympathy and attention from outsiders, who always think that the trouble has been contracted in the discharge of her duties and, therefore, regard her as a martyr. But in the majority of these cases, the superintendent, not wishing to be misunderstood, or to be regarded as altogether heartless, keeps her own counsel, otherwise she would explain that the pupil's work has had little or nothing to do with her sickness, which, on the contrary, has been due to pure thoughtlessness or carelessness on her part. For this reason alone superintendents would find it advisable to choose, out of the numerous candidates who present themselves, women of mature experience and not young, heedless, giddy girls, who are worse than children in the matter of extra care that often has to be bestowed upon them.

Any nurse who will feign illness for the sake of a little rest, or from natural indolence, cannot be too severely censured, and the sooner the school is rid of her presence, the better; good time and training should not be wasted upon anyone who develops such evidence of a total lack of honor and honesty.

In order, then, that a nurse may keep her health with a fair amount of certainty, unless the unforeseen occurs, she must understand, and intelligently conform to, certain cardinal laws. Of these the most important are cleanliness in regard to her person, and systematic, regular habits as regards eating, sleeping, exercise and recreation. But let her also remember that all extremes are bad and that she must not degenerate into a fussy valetudinarian. After giving proper attention to her body in these respects, let her stop thinking about it and it will very well take care of itself. Ill effects will almost inevitably result from allowing the mind to dwell too much upon the body. Here, as elsewhere, moderation and common-sense are indispensable, if we would maintain a condition of mind that will have no room in it for the development of imaginary pains or diseases. In addition to the broad laws of health, there are certain minor points that from the nature of her work, a nurse should strictly observe. With these, therefore, we shall deal somewhat in detail.

General *personal cleanliness* means a plentiful use of water in order to keep the skin fresh, clean and clear looking, to remove the impurities that have collected upon it, both from within and without, and to keep it active so that it can do its work unhampered. A full warm (not hot) bath once a day is highly desirable. This acts best when taken at night before going to bed, as it helps to relax the tension of nerves and muscles and in most people induces sleep, not to mention the fact that sudden exposures to extreme variations in temperature, which often lead to the development of sore-throats or colds, are also avoided. The morning bath should be nothing more than a quick, cold or tepid, sponge with a brisk rubbing, which leaves one feeling wide awake, in good spirits and in an equable temper, ready to begin the day's work. Judgment must be exercised in bathing, as in everything else; it can be overdone, and what may benefit one woman may result in much harm to another, whose powers of reaction are not so vigorous. I have known not a few people, who bathed too much, to suffer in consequence from a nervous, depressed condition and indigestion. A warm tub-bath twice a day is inadvisable for anyone, and sometimes it may be best to take it only once a week, confining oneself, as a rule, on the other days, to the sponge and rub. Remaining too long in warm or cold water should always be avoided.

In a hospital the nurse's *hair* requires more frequent washing than at home, since the dust, which it catches, is more liable to contain germs of disease. An abundant head of hair will often absorb disagreeable odors, if the owner has to remain long in an atmosphere laden with impurities, as for instance, when dressing certain kinds of surgical wounds or in dispensary work) It should, therefore, be washed about every two weeks, with warm water and soap, or with water containing a little borax, being afterwards dried in the sun-shine. In training schools there are usually certain regulations dealing with the dressing of the hair with which a junior nurse should readily comply, even if the style is not always agreeable to her. Thus, a usual requirement is that the hair shall be dressed in a simple manner and worn off the face. Nor is this a purely arbitrary regulation, since an elaborately arranged coiffure mean the devotion of a good deal of time to it, which a busy nurse can ill afford, and because a simple, neat style is more in keeping with the work and uniform, while it lends dignity to the personal appearance. Again, the hair ought to be brushed off the face for two reasons; first, because curls or bangs require special attention to make them really becoming, and secondly, any fringe or loose ends of hair, falling around the face or about the head, may prove a source of infection to patients, for the reason that such locks readily catch dust particles, which may be readily scattered from them upon wounds and dressings. It is not necessary to have the hair drawn back so tightly that it is unbecoming; it can be brushed to roll back in a soft natural way that is far more attractive than many of the other styles affected.

It would hardly seem necessary to dwell upon the special care that should be given to the *teeth* and to the *breath,* had not some of us painful recollections of good nurses and really nice, lovable women, whose negligence in the care of their teeth and the disagreeable odor of whose breath were conspicuous. Some teeth will never look pretty, but at least, one can make sure they are absolutely clean and that particles of food are not clinging to them. Vigorous brushing with a good soap and fresh water after meals, together with the habitual use of dental silk, and an occasional visit to the dentist, will keep any teeth clean and fresh looking.

Under no circumstances should a nurse with a foul breath work over a patient. This defect may come from decayed teeth, or be the result of a disordered stomach, or of a catarrhal condition of the throat or nose. If dieting and attention to the bowels do not improve the digestion, the superintendent of nurses should be told and a physician should be consulted. A chronic catarrh of the nose or throat disqualifies a woman for nursing for many reasons. Any chronic inflammation or discharge from any organ of the body may be not only a source of bad odors, but also a cause of infection to wounds with which she may have to deal. As was said before, a sick person's senses are often abnormally acute, and any foul smell would prove a source of unpleasantness even to the verge of nausea. The same may be said of the odor from the sweat glands in the axillae. A woman who perspires very readily must be exceedingly careful that no odor is ever perceptible. If this *excessive perspiration* be beyond her control — as is sometimes the case — a dermatologist should be consulted. Frequently, however, it has to be regarded as a form of nervousness and can then be checked, partially at least, by trying to preserve a more equable temperament. Careful and frequent bathing with soap and water is always necessary, followed by the use of talcum or of plain rice powder of a good quality.

Under no circumstances should a nurse indulge in the use of *perfumes* either upon her person or clothes. Their employment is evidence of a certain vulgarity at any time and, in the case of nurses, is usually looked upon with suspicion, as a slipshod way of concealing uncleanliness. Apart from all this, she owes it to her patients to be on the safe side in this respect. People differ so greatly in the matter of perfumes that what to one may be a most agreeable scent, to another may be extremely obnoxious. In fact I have known patients who have suffered from a sensation of nausea due to perfume worn by the nurse, and yet have been very unwilling to make any objection from fear of hurting her feelings.

In the course of her training, a nurse will learn the various sources of infection and the important part the *hands* may play in propagating various morbid processes. (From the very beginning, as a habit of vital importance in connection with the care of her health, she must learn never to touch her face, her eyes, or lips, with her hands, unless she is sure they are perfectly clean and free from infectious material, and never to put pins in her mouth. Some of the cases of typhoid fever contracted by nurses, while caring for individuals suffering with this disease, might have been avoided had each nurse always remembered the precaution never to touch her face with her hands, while working over her patients, and never to partake of food until her hands had been thoroughly disinfected. Again, after one patient has been cared for, the nurse should always scrub her hands before going to the next. For this reason, and because it has a dainty look in the eyes of the patient, she should make a practice of always washing her hands before handling his food or preparing his medicine. As far as possible, the use of the handkerchief should be avoided, especially when working over wounds, preparing dressings, or assisting at operations. The nurse should be particularly careful never to rub her eye or to allow any discharges to get into it. If, however, such an accident happens, she should seek proper treatment at once, since the resulting infection may give a great deal of trouble and might even result in the loss of sight. Little cuts and scratches should never be neglected, as one can readily become infected after the skin is broken. Apparently trivial injuries inflicted by a pin in a dressing on a patient have been known to set up inflammatory processes necessitating quite grave operations. A nurse receiving such a wound, however small it may be, should squeeze the place hard enough to make it bleed freely, and then wash the part with very hot water and keep it covered. Be careful not to bandage the wound too tightly and never use a rubber band, which will interfere with the circulation. If the part becomes red and painful, put on a hot wet boracic acid dressing and report the matter at once. Any cuts about the hands, or sores under the fingernails, should be shown to the head-nurse at once — not two or three days after they have begun to be painful. By obtaining good advice and prompt treatment, much suffering, loss of time, and perhaps an operation may be avoided. Processes around or under the nails are apt to be very virulent. To get rid of infectious material, the hands and nails should be frequently scrubbed with warm water and soap, a good stiff brush being employed. This brush should be kept in a solution of 1-40 carbolic acid. If too stiff and used too vigorously, however, it may wound the tender cuticle under the nail and thus increase the danger of infection. Nurses in operating-rooms, in particular, should bear this in mind.

Constant washing and the use of disinfectant solutions at first will often irritate the soft skin of the hands, making them rough to the touch. Whenever they become chapped, they will require special attention and it will be advisable to wrap them at night in a dressing, to which some bland healing ointment has been applied. To avoid this chapping and roughness, the nurse should be very careful always to thoroughly dry her hands after each washing, since it is important that they should always be as soft, smooth and attractive looking as circumstances will permit. The nature of the work will sometimes prevent them from appearing very white, but at least they should show signs of being well kept. Fashionably pointed, brilliantly polished and tinted finger-nails are not in good taste any more than an extreme mode in dressing the hair. The nails should be filed as short as possible, to prevent the accumulation under them of any dirt, that may contain infectious germs, and to avoid any risk of scratching the patient. Sometimes nurses are troubled with very cold or hot, feverish hands, or, worse than all, with clammy, nervous hands that have a chilling touch. Cold hands may sometimes be benefited by wearing extra under-flannels, and thus assisting the circulation in them. Cooling lotions may improve the hot, feverish hand, although, as in the case of the nervous, clammy hand, no doubt systematic treatment might do more, by bringing the general nervous system into better order. So far as regards local treatment, an alcohol rub and rice powder, applied just before touching the patient will help for the moment. With such hands, unless one is obliged to rub the patient, it is best, as far as possible, to avoid touching her. After giving your hands the proper care, let them alone; never make them an object of special study or gaze admiringly at them in the presence of the patient.

The *foot* is a part of the anatomy that demands the attention of at least three-fourths of the women who take up hospital life. The nurse is fortunate, indeed, who escapes trouble with her feet. The mischief is largely caused by the unusual strain of having to be on one's feet for so long a time at a stretch, to the constant walking to and fro on hard polished floors, to the extra strain a new nurse puts on them in her efforts to move quietly without making a noise, but, above all, to the defective style of shoe generally worn. To avoid this painful condition, a new nurse should first supply herself with a comfortable, not too loose-fitting, shoe; it should be tight enough to hold her foot snugly, but should not pinch at any point; it should also give sufficient support to the instep and ankle. It should be broad enough to allow free movement to the toes, and just high enough at the heel to prevent the wearer from dropping back when walking, while not tipping forward towards the toes. It would be ridiculous to attempt to prescribe any one particular style of shoe and expect all kinds of feet to be comfortable in it. The characteristics of the individual foot must be taken into consideration. The feet should be bathed every day in tepid water and vigorously rubbed; the stockings should be changed frequently and no special effort should be made to walk noiselessly. To overcome any difficulty in this respect, and in order to enable the wearer to move quietly, a small rubber plate may be attached to the heel of the shoe. All squeaking shoes should be discarded at once. All-rubber soles should not be worn, as they tend to aggravate the soreness. Before being accepted, probationers should have their feet examined. A woman with a marked flat-foot should be rejected, as in almost every instance such a defect will sooner or later compel her to give up her work or else to undergo much suffering. A tendency to flat-footedness may not be detected until after the pupil has been in training for a year or more. When discovered, the condition should at once be reported by the superintendent to the surgeon, who may be able to overcome it by a specially devised shoe, or by other methods. Slippers should not be worn at any time, either on day or night duty, or in private houses. They are apt to cause swelling of the ankles if the nurse is on her feet for any great length of time; they offer no support to the instep or ankles and unnecessarily hasten a feeling of fatigue.

Cleanliness, then is all important, but in order to preserve vigor, strength and harmony in the whole body, regularity in eating, sleeping, exercise and recreation is also necessary. No human being — least of all a nurse — can with impunity disregard regularity of habits in respect to these vital factors in the preservation of health.

In the matter of *food* too much stress cannot be laid upon the importance of not permitting any license in regard to eating out of meal hours. Particularly pernicious is the habit of having suppers night after night, first in one nurse's room and then in another's. Such indulgence is too apt to lead to dissipation in other ways as well, remaining up too late, gossiping, the needless expenditure of money, rising late the next morning, which entails a hurried half-made toilet, a half-tidied room and no appetite for breakfast. No wonder that the work in the ward drags; no wonder that there are listlessness and a lack of energy and interest — all of which have their effect upon the patients. Make it a habit to rise instantly the dressing bell rings, so as to have plenty of time to dress, to leave your room and bed in condition for proper airing, and to be punctual at the breakfast table, where a good plain substantial meal ought to be taken with a relish and without haste. A nurse who would rather go without her breakfast is in no condition to go into the wards of a hospital to work over sick people, for without proper food, the bodily resistance is lowered and she is, therefore, much more susceptible to disease. A cup of tea or coffee is not sufficient; it may supply a stimulus which will enable one to keep up for the time being at the expense of pure nerve force; but sooner or later the system will show the effect of such maltreatment. The nurse, who has taken no breakfast, about ten or eleven o'clock begins to feel the effect of the want of food and goes to the ward kitchen and partakes of milk, bread and butter, or whatever she may find at hand. In this she is doing wrong in two ways. The food is not hers; it has been provided for the patients, and although there may be plenty for all, the principle is absolutely wrong. As the caretaker of the patients and all that belongs to them, she has no right at any time to appropriate their property. If she permits herself such liberties, her character and ideals suffer in consequence. Secondly, when dinner-time comes she has no appetite and, instead of blaming herself, she is apt to criticize the food, and thus encourage in herself and others the habit of fault-finding and grumbling.

The food supplied for hospital workers should be of the best quality, plain, wholesome and abundant, well cooked, attractively served, and with sufficient variety to break the monotony. I am afraid that some hospital boards display a somewhat short-sighted policy in this respect; since a plain but liberal diet for the nurses is amply repaid by the better nursing accomplished.

But even if she has every opportunity of exceeding, a nurse should always be strictly temperate in eating. Indiscretion in diet always has a bad effect, making one irritable, cross and exacting. Any irregularity of the bowels, either in the way of constipation or diarrhoea, should never be neglected. As a preventive or as a curative measure, a proper diet is all important. A nurse must not get into the habit of depending upon medicines for constipation and a woman who is suffering from diarrhoea ought to have will-power and sense enough to restrict herself in the kinds of food she takes. Such thoughtlessness and want of sense do not seem possible, but it not infrequently happens that a woman will wonder why the medicine provided for her does not seem to do her any good, while in the meantime her diet is aggravating the disease.

But when a nurse is suffering from indigestion, depression or extra fatigue, no matter from what cause, let her be very careful not to attempt to build up her flagging energies by excessive quantities of tea and coffee. The abuse of such stimulants will only aggravate the trouble and in the end leave her with the tea and coffee habit. Remember that tea and coffee are really drugs and their excessive use is a form of dissipation removed only in degree from that of alcohol or narcotics. It would seem hardly necessary to say that under no circumstances should a nurse ever allow herself to take an alcoholic stimulant or any narcotic or anodyne, unless by the express order from the physician conveyed through the superintendent of the school. But since she has every opportunity of obtaining them, she must steadfastly resolve never to touch them, even in the way of experiment and in order to test their effect. Among my saddest experiences are the instances, fortunately very rare, in which I have encountered members of our profession, who have lost their power of self-control and have become victims to the abuse of some powerful drug or alcoholic stimulant with all its attending evils.

Sleep and recreation are the two great natural correctives for mental and physical wear and tear. It is wonderful how large an amount of physical exertion can be borne without injury to the health, provided that sufficient and regular hours for sleep are obtained. The proper amount of sleep is necessary more especially for the junior nurse. For the first few weeks or months of her training, she is under an unusual physical and mental strain; and until she has had time to adjust herself, as it were, to the demands made upon her mind and body, she needs at least eight consecutive hours of sleep, although later on she may be able to do with less. It is, therefore, no arbitrary school rule that requires lights to be out at ten o'clock when the dressing bell rings at six in the morning. Nor should pleasure, study, or the love of social intercourse with her fellow-workers, prevent a nurse from adhering to this rule. During the time that she is off duty in the daytime, it is a good plan to lie down for a half hour to relax both nerve and muscle tension, and then go out in the fresh air for another half hour, if only to take a turn around the square, or a street-car ride. The change of scene and air and the increased supply of oxygen in the system will help her to throw off any feeling of languor and depression, and she will return to her work with renewed energy, feeling refreshed and bright.

A regular amount of well-ordered *recreation* is just as necessary for the health as food and sleep, and the very nature of nursing work demands a frequent change of atmosphere and thought. Only she must be careful to decide wisely just where recreation ends and dissipation begins. She should systematically plan to get right away from the hospital once a week, to free herself from all thoughts about nursing for the time and enjoy herself according to her own tastes. Thus, once a week she may dine or sup with friends, hear a good concert or see a good play, take a run out into the country, or visit a picture-gallery, spending as little time as possible in crowded and ill-ventilated shops. On one day out of seven, then, she should devote several consecutive hours to pure recreation. With the hours taken up in study, ward-work, classes and lectures and in getting the necessary amount of sleep, more than this is not possible, without over-taxing one's energies or neglecting one's studies or duties. Whenever possible, a part of every Sunday should be devoted to religious duties and the nurse should plan to attend church service either in the morning or evening. There is, of course, a great temptation to spend her spare time in resting or reading, but a little thought will show her that the spiritual side of a nurse's nature needs the opportunity for real rest — away from the world — and quiet meditation afforded by the hour in church, while in the end the extra effort will strengthen the moral character and lead to the formation of a desirable habit.

The length of the annual vacation is usually set at two weeks, but occasionally a pupil-nurse may wish to shorten her time in the school by giving up her vacation; or at other times she may ask for four weeks one year, leaving no time for the next. After years of observation I am convinced that both plans are false economy, and I am sure that, in the best interests of the nurse, all schools should arrange to have the two weeks' holiday obligatory. Without even this brief period of absolute rest, change and recreation, there is apt to be a marked difference in the character and spirit of the work done during the next year; more effort will be required to accomplish it, and in some cases the nurse will break down and in the end lose more time than she tried to save. Each year requires its own share of freedom from duty, if a nurse would do good work in the right spirit and preserve her health; and to utilize this vacation for true recreation, a woman should leave her work behind her and surround herself with quite different thoughts and scenes, not indeed entering upon a round of ceaseless gaiety, but obtaining a happy mixture of rest and pleasure. But the cultivation of this habit of laying aside her cares should apply equally to the work of every day. When a nurse leaves the ward, she should cease to dwell upon what has happened or is about to happen in it; she should not waste time in continually talking over the day's doings with others and in morbidly refusing to think of anything else. The nurse who takes the best care of her patients, and whose personality is the most attractive to them, is not apt to be one who allows herself to get into such a narrow way of thinking. When with her patients she should be devotion itself, but when she leaves them, she should divert her mind to other things and so bring back with her on her return a fresh breath of the outside world, which stirs their pulses, makes them forget themselves for the moment and gives them a stronger desire to get well. Good normal health does not permit of anything in the way of morbidness; it demands the natural stimulus of change of air, scene and thought.

Finally, the body should be *properly clothed* against sudden changes of temperature, which can scarcely be avoided. The uniform, which is always of some light cotton material, affords no protection against cold draughty corridors, which a nurse may have to pass through, after becoming over-heated at her work in the wards or in the operating-room. Such exposure may be followed by sore-throat, rheumatism, or a heavy cold, unless proper precautions are taken. It is highly desirable, then, to always wear appropriate underclothing, which in winter should be warm, but not too heavy in weight. The chest, arms and feet should be well covered; a long-sleeved, high-necked undergarment should always be worn in winter. I have known several instances in which rheumatism developed, when this precaution had been neglected. Every article of clothing worn by a nurse, when busied with the sick, should be of washing material. It is pleasant to think how absolutely clean and at the same time how dainty an appearance a nurse can present at a comparatively small cost. Everything she wears should bear the stamp of simplicity and refinement upon it. Embroideries and laces, ruffles and frills, are out of place upon her under-garments, because she no longer has the time to keep in proper repair such elaborate trimmings; and besides in no institution laundry would it be possible to allow the attention requisite for washing and ironing fine clothes. Be assured that a woman shows good judgment and better taste, when she folds away her finery for her holiday season and furnishes herself with a wardrobe of plain, substantial underclothing, which should be changed frequently enough to keep it fresh and free from odor.

And lastly, since the nurse's external surroundings are apt to bear an important relation to her health, she should take particular care that her *sleeping-room* is arranged properly and with due regard to the laws of hygiene. It is now a rare occurrence to find a school for nurses that is not amply, if not luxuriously, supplied with reception and sitting rooms, and that has not a library study for the use of its students. It is, therefore, no longer necessary for the nurse to convert her one small bed-room into an attempted combination of all these. On the contrary, for many reasons, its arrangement should be almost severe in its simplicity, while from a hygienic standpoint it is desirable to have as little furniture as possible. An accumulation of all kinds of odds and ends, tacked up on the walls, a number of cheap hangings, coverings and cushions, occupying every spare inch of space, are just so many dust catchers, and plenty of good time and strength must be sacrificed if they are to be kept clean and attractive. Furthermore, any attempt at ornamentation with cheap materials will probably not be in the best of taste, and it is far better to be content with a small amount of something really good of its kind. A nurse has no longer the time to take care of an overcrowded sleeping-room, and furthermore, she owes it to her nerves to lie down to rest in a room that does not jar upon them with a sense of confusion. She should, therefore, regard her sleeping-room as essentially a place for wholesome rest and give it a liberal supply of fresh air and all the sunshine available. The furniture should be sufficiently simple so that it will be always possible to keep it absolutely clean and orderly, with a minimum expenditure of time and strength. Nothing in the way of soiled clothing should be allowed to lie about; all vessels should be kept sweet and clean, even if this has to be attended to by the nurse herself. In all kinds of weather she should sleep with her window sufficiently wide open to allow of free ventilation, and it should be her daily practice to thoroughly open up her bed to air, beating up the pillows, throwing back the coverings separately and in such a way as not to touch the floor, and turning up the mattress. The appearance of a nurse's room and the care she gives it are additional means of judging of the character of the occupant.

Chapter Seven - Uniform - Dress - Economy

Every training school requires that the pupils shall wear the *uniform* prescribed by the authorities. In former days each nurse was expected to provide her own dresses, with the result that incongruities were often met with. But in those institutions which have taken upon themselves to supervise and be responsible for the making of all uniforms, we are more apt to find the dresses as they should be, with the same style and cut of -sleeves and waist, the same length of apron, the same depth of hem, and the same general trigness throughout, not to mention a conspicuous and pleasing absence of extraneous ornamentation of any kind. Provided with a generous outfit of uniforms and accorded the privilege of the laundry, it would hardly seem possible that a pupil-nurse could ever present other than a neat, clean appearance, or that at the end of her time she could be otherwise than steeped in the principles and practice of personal neatness and cleanliness. But even after starting aright, good habits are not formed in a day, and unless strict attention is paid to details in the matter of fresh collars and cuffs, a clean uncrumpled dress and apron, to buttons all occupying their proper places, and not giving way to safety pins, to nicely arranged hair and neatly dressed feet, a woman, in spite of her uniform, can present an untidy, careless appearance, which detracts very greatly from her personality, and which justifies a suspicion that she may carry this looseness in the matter of details into all her work. Perhaps the most serious drawback to uniforms of the present day lies in the fact that they are done up with too much starch and in consequence are a source of annoyance to both wearer and patient, owing to the rustling and crackling which follow every movement of the nurse, until the dress loses its stiffness and hangs soft and limp. Of course the starch is employed as a means of saving, since it keeps the uniform fresh-looking longer, but it is high time that institutions recognized the fact that true economy can never be attained by the sacrifice of a principle. No clothing is suitable for a woman, who is in attendance upon the sick and nervous, that will not permit her to move with perfect freedom and yet noiselessly. Cuffs that are shorty stiff and starched like boards, should never form a part of a nurse's uniform. It is true they may serve as a finish to her costume, but they afford no protection for her dress-sleeves, and, moreover, in working about her patient, the sharp edges are more than likely to hurt some part of the body by coming sharply in contact with it. On the other hand, a cuff made of soft plain cambric, and reaching to the elbow, looks equally neat, and at the same time will effectually protect the sleeve of the dress. Moreover, it is easily washed, and thus can be frequently changed with but little expense, and is readily removed before meals. There is still much to be desired in regard to the cap, not only in the making, but also in the wearing. It is rare to find the various members of any school with caps that seem to be a part of a set uniform, and the reckless, flyaway fashion, in which these are frequently carried on the head, furnishes food for thought in regard to the wearers. Formerly, caps were worn in order to protect the hair from dust and as a badge of servitude. Now-a-days, they can scarcely be regarded as more than a finish to a nurse's costume, holding a place similar to that of the mortar-board as regards the college student's gown.

Of the times when the uniform has its objections, something will be said in the chapter on private duty, but from the outset a young nurse should give due consideration to her uniform and to its various possible uses and abuses. That the wearing of it in a hospital marks and sets her apart from other classes of workers about the place, and that it inspires her patients with confidence and commands an added respect from all, there is no question. On the other hand, its wearer should always remember that it should be held in proper regard and kept sacred, as it were, to the particular work for which it was designed, lest by any act of hers its dignity become impaired. A nurse, therefore, is never allowed to appear in the wards of the hospital in any costume except her uniform. Nor should the latter ever be made to do duty as a walking dress, for that would be to render it conspicuous and attract undesirable and unnecessary attention from the public. Nor should it be worn to places of amusement, where it might unseasonably emphasize the nearness of sickness and death. It is, therefore, inappropriate for a nurse to appear in her uniform at all times and in all places, when she is off duty, and in this matter, as well as in other respects, she is expected to show her appreciation of the fitness of things, which can be evidenced by her *civilian dress* no less than by her uniform. In her capacity as a nurse, it is not seemly that she should have ambitions to appear as "the glass of fashion, or the mould of form." Even when she is a woman of independent means and the matter of expense does not enter into the question, she is not justified in appearing in raiment other than that becoming her vocation. A woman's character is estimated by the way in which she dresses, as well as by her manners, and a nurse's costume should at all times be characterized by a certain quiet good taste, as regards both colors and style, while at the same time giving the impression that she is well dressed. Her wardrobe need never be very extensive; a good tailor-made walking or travelling dress, a house dress and a pretty dinner or evening dress are all that are necessary at any time in addition to her uniform. As she intends to continue in her style of dress, so should she begin, for there are other and better ways in which to spend her superfluous energy and money than in trying to keep up with the latest style in dress. On the other hand, a nurse cannot afford to affect peculiarities, or show too great an indifference to her appearance, and go about in ill-fitting, ill-selected, shabby gowns, that a respectable servant-maid would not think of wearing. Both extremes are bad, and here, as in other things, the golden mean should be cultivated.

There is another important reason why she should place a limit upon the quality and quantity of her wardrobe, namely, because moderation in this respect affords a splendid opportunity for the exercise of *economy*. This virtue, so rarely found and yet so important for women to whose charge is entrusted the property of others as well as their own, is deserving of much more attention in training schools than it receives at present. A special course should be devoted to this subject, and it should be taught both from a theoretical and from a practical standpoint. In the hospital the nurse will have many opportunities for practising economy, until the exercise of it becomes a second nature. It is a common experience to find individuals, —that are wantonly extravagant with other people's property, positively stingy where their own is concerned. But whether a thing belongs to you, or to someone else, need not enter into consideration. Carefulness should be exercised on principle, because it is wrong to be wasteful. Unfortunately, nurses often become too familiar with extravagance in their hospital life, on account of the example set them by some of the physicians in their lavish use of dressing materials, in the careless ordering of needlessly large quantities of expensive drugs, and in the want of care shown in dealing with instruments and hospital materials in general. But this should not make the nurse less guarded, or less interested in trying to show her appreciation of the value of the things she has to work with.

It would hardly seem necessary to mention the many temptations to carelessness and *extravagance*. Linen of all kinds may be used unnecessarily; sheets and towels and clothing may be changed, when hardly soiled, or when a little judicious management would effect equally good results; or again, linen may be stained and spoiled merely because the nurse has not been careful to protect it properly from dressings or drugs. The exchange list at the end of the month will testify to such carelessness, when linen has to be discarded, not because it is worn out, but because it is too unsightly for use on account of the stains upon it. Even expensive flannel blankets do not always meet with respect, and a heedless junior may pull down the finest, best blanket, in which to wrap a patient covered with burns and grease, when an older one — softer and much more appropriate, although less valuable — is near at hand. Again, in the matter of food, not even a slice of bread should be wasted unnecessarily; and the same rule applies to the use of solutions, alcohol, gas, and even of pins, needles and the like. For keeping up the supply of rubber applications alone — hot-water bags, rubber-sheets, syringes, etc. — the expense is enormous, while the breakage in thermometers in the course of a year is more than the cost of several patients. Again, experience has shown that the list of broken china is far too long, even when a check is put upon it by requiring that all articles shall be replaced. A nurse should use her ingenuity and plan to do just as good work with a limited supply as ordinary people would do with double the quantity. It should be a matter of pride with her to make the most of everything. These are some of the ways in which she can show the good results of her training, and which should render her work of more value than that of the well-meaning amateur. She should do more and better with less appliances and at less expense to either the hospital or the home. When one takes into consideration the cost for a year of the combined waste in a school of seventy or eighty women, and then calculates what a reduction might be effected, if each one would exercise only ordinary care and economy, it will readily be seen that the results would contribute considerably to the usefulness of the hospital, inasmuch as a greater number of patients could be cared for at the same cost. Let the nurse, then, remember that she contributes to charity just in proportion as she exercises thrift and economy in the care she takes of the materials with which she is entrusted.

In our modern hospitals it would almost seem as though things were made too easy and too many tools were supplied to work with, thus doing away with the necessity for invention and for devising ways and means that formed so valuable a part of the training in the earlier days.

Economy of time is also no small item in the course of a three years' training. A woman should be careful how she expends it both on and off duty. She should not allow her free hours to be absorbed by other people to such an extent as to interfere with study, sleep, or recreation. Again, she should have the courage and good sense to refuse to spend her money on unnecessary luxuries in the way of food, frequent dinners at some expensive hotel, late suppers, candy, etc. All such doings are liable to lead to the formation of habits of extravagance and after a while one's nature refuses to find satisfaction in the simple pleasures and simple living, which should mark the life of a nurse. Ease, luxury and self-indulgence are not compatible with true devotion to nursing work, and it is best not to begin by permitting oneself any latitude in this respect.

It is generally said of nurses that they are unbusinesslike — a grave criticism, indeed, on women who should be remarkable for their prudence and practical methods, for their careful ordering, thrift and discretion, as evidenced alike in their manner of work and personality. The systematic training in due carefulness, economy and in counting the cost of one's various expenditures during one's time in the hospital, will enable a woman to enter upon her work as a private nurse, prepared to be an economical factor in the true sense, when she goes into a family, instead of adding to the reputation for extravagance that nurses have succeeded in acquiring, and which, in some instances, no doubt is deserved. It may be said that a nurse should not be criticized too sharply, since she can hardly be regarded as an exception in these days, when the desire for creature comforts and luxuries is so rampant in the land; when extravagance abounds on every hand and the qualities of thrift and high thinking and simple living are at so great a discount. But perhaps she is the less to be excused because, touching as she does the extremes of living both in her hospital and private practice, she should learn the lesson that the happy mean is found in the life that offers neither poverty nor riches; and because it is her duty to educate others in this respect, both by example and precept. Such habits of mind, of body, and of good economics, however, can be acquired only by a regular and systematic cultivation of them. This means that the principles of method, order and system should be carried into everything a nurse does, and diligently practised, until finally they become a matter of routine and part of her nature.

To all the other good habits there remains to be added *studiousness*. With the present graded system of class instruction, lectures and demonstrations, a pupil is obliged to do a certain amount of study, if she wishes to pass her examinations and obtain her certificate. With this obligatory minimum she is too apt to be satisfied, unless she has learned to love knowledge for its own sake and to appreciate its importance. Systematic study is the only method of acquiring and satisfying this desire for further knowledge and of developing opportunities. In order to begin the formation of studious habits, the junior nurse should pay strict attention to the prescribed subjects; the time for reading and studying should be as regularly observed as the hour for going on duty at the hospital; her classwork and lectures should be prepared gradually, day by day. Method is all-important. A hurried hour snatched on the day before, or perhaps on the very day of, the class recitation will not answer the purpose. Nor is it wise for her to devote the greater portion of the Sunday's leisure hours to catching up with her tasks and thus depriving herself of her proper amount of rest and recreation. It is true that with this apology for study she may pass muster, although she will probably stand low in her class and get through with a question mark after her name, but to the end any information, that she may gain, will be of the most superficial character, not to be depended upon and likely to fail her utterly in the hour of emergency, when only the right kind of knowledge will fit the occasion. Nor will it be such as is calculated to increase her self-reliance and enable her to think and act for herself. "If a thing is worth doing at all, it is worth doing well" applies very well to nursing; and if a woman makes this her profession, she should be satisfied with nothing else than being a first-rate nurse — not second-rate, average or mediocre, but the best that willingness, intelligence and application can make her. Study to such a woman will gradually take in other subjects besides those that are obligatory and prescribed. Her attitude of mind and desire for knowledge will help to develop her powers of observation, and acuteness of perception; and as she goes about her work, all that happens around her will have a new and interesting meaning for her and she will gradually develop a genuine habit of study. The habit of reasoning and pondering over the meaning and application of principles will result in her work being done with more thoroughness, energy and intelligence, and the hard, matter-of-fact duties will be cheerfully performed, in the light of the deep significance which lies behind them. Nor will she be content to accept present knowledge alone; she will want to know about the older methods of doing things, will make comparisons and deductions, and as a result may be able to add some improvement to existing methods and so make the work that much better. Such a student will always keep her mind open to receive instruction from all sources and without prejudice, and will not hesitate to modify her views, whenever it is necessary to do so, in order to keep pace with the newer developments and continual progress, that is so marked a feature of the medical profession of the present day. The obligatory instruction should, therefore, be regarded as affording opportunities to start one on the right road to self-imposed study, and not merely as a hard, disagreeable task, the sooner done with the better.

A woman of educated intelligence will naturally bring to the study of nursing an ease and readiness of application unknown to those whose intellects have remained untrained. Moreover, she is at a distinct advantage, inasmuch as she can, at the same time, readily keep up her general reading and information. If she has once reached a certain point, she will never allow herself to rest upon general knowledge already acquired, or to grow rusty in this respect, recognizing the fact that her technical knowledge and skill represent only part of what her attainments should be, for her ministrations must often be directed to a diseased mind rather than to a sick body. In such cases her practical manual dexterity will be less useful and important than the skilful use of her ethical qualities and of her general knowledge. Frequently she will meet with the stage in recovery, when to be able to amuse, entertain, read aloud well, or even turn her hands to account, are the best and most acceptable form of medicine in hastening the patient's recovery. Any nurse, who fails to cultivate this form of study and knowledge, will be sure to have a too pronounced professional attitude, and be too limited in her resources to be a thorough success. Finally, it must be remembered that professional and general knowledge should be kept modestly in the background; they should be brought out only to meet the proper occasions and should never be put on parade, just for the sake of making an impression as a clever or learned person.

Chapter Eight - Night-Duty

When detailed for night-duty, the junior nurse takes the first step in actual serious responsibility in her career. Once she has passed this first crucial test, her responsibilities progressively increase through the various stages of intermediate and senior work, until finally, if she has displayed the requisite ability in meeting them, she becomes qualified for the most important post of all - that of head-nurse of a ward. A junior nurse is not put on her first night-duty until she has already passed through about four months of training. She has, therefore, had time to learn the first principles of her practical work, which she will now be expected to apply on her own responsibility and without having her head-nurse, or some other older nurse, constantly at her elbow to observe, direct, assist or encourage her. Night-duty is also a wonderful test of the ethical side of nursing. It touches it at almost every point and brings out the weak and strong points in a woman's character. The nurse should, therefore, bear in mind that it affords opportunities for the development of such characteristics as will strengthen the moral side of her nature. There is no better time for learning to develop self-dependence, self-control and good judgment. To be sure, she always has the privilege of calling upon the night head-nurse for advice and help in untried situations, but it is not desirable to make too frequent appeals, and she therefore displays her judgment, in knowing when to have recourse to such help, and in proving that she can distinguish between grave and trivial situations. Above all, night-duty is an admirable test as to the amount of forethought and system that she possesses. The former is necessary for planning out work and keeping ahead of it, while a thorough system will enable her to do, in the best way, the greatest possible amount of work in the least possible time; and both those qualities must be put into execution, if she is to make a reputation for good night work. For ten or twelve hours of the night, the ward and its patients are in her keeping and the degree of care they receive must depend upon her capacity. She has now to do more with pure nursing and comes in more personal relations with the patients than she did when on day-duty. At the same time she is expected to take proper care of the various appliances, with, which she works, and to leave them, as well as the ward generally, in proper order before going off duty in the morning. She has to learn to arrange matters so as not to spend so much time over one patient, or piece of work, that the rest are neglected. Orders must be carried out punctually; prescribed medicines and nourishment must be given at the exact hour named — not even ten minutes before or after; temperatures and pulses must be taken in the same punctual way; everything must be done on time, and when some grave emergency interferes, any discrepancy should be reported to the proper authorities. It is never allowable in a nurse to be unpunctual in the carrying out of orders. Night duty, therefore, puts to the test her honor and honesty, since there is no one always at hand to watch her and see that she performs conscientiously every duty required of her; that she never records anything in the way of temperatures, medicines given, or treatment, that is not strictly true. Her aim should be to try and be a little more faithful, a little more accurate, if possible, in carrying out her duties when alone than when under observation.

The night-nurse not infrequently has opportunities of testing her presence of mind, and of bringing into action her resources, since she is liable to have to deal with emergencies of various kinds. Probably there are few demands she will ever have to meet that will try her courage in the same way as her first night-work, with its new and unexpected possibilities. But such a test has its rewards as well, for it will leave her with a feeling of self-reliance and experience that no other form of the nursing can supply so well and at so fitting a time.

A night-nurse reports for duty to the night head-nurse, as punctually at the hour for going on as when on day duty. After reaching the ward, she should go directly to her head-nurse, or whoever is in charge, for her night orders, which she will find written out and which she reads over carefully. In addition, she receives an account of any changes that may have taken place during the day in any of the patients, and special directions with regard to new patients, who have come in as well as to any other matters of importance. She may ask any questions, until she is quite certain that she understands what is expected of her, and then, without further words or loss of time, she should quietly proceed with her work. Lights in hospital wards are, as a rule, turned down at nine o'clock, and for this reason she tries to get any work, that requires much walking about, finished before that time. She should make it a point to pay a brief visit to each patient, to judge for herself of the condition of the old ones and to give each a pleasant little greeting, as well as to make the acquaintance of any newcomers and to put them at their ease. The turning down of the lights should always be an indication that all noise must cease in or about the ward. A good night-nurse never permits anyone to transgress this rule; she herself sets an example by perfect quietness in her actions, moving about noiselessly as though shod with velvet. The necessary reports to the physician and night-head-nurse should be made distinctly but not in tones loud enough to disturb the patients. Laughing and talking are out of place, and any disposition on the part of the doctor to stop for a friendly chat should be emphatically discouraged. Such visits naturally take time and interfere with the work; they also lay the nurse open to criticism from the patients. Thus, if she is the only woman in a ward full of men, and if the doctor makes frequent visits and prolongs his stay, talking with the nurse, the latter will inevitably run the risk of losing, in some measure, the respect and high regard in which the patients should hold her, while at the same time the dignity of her position suffers in consequence. The patients in the free wards naturally take their tone at night from the woman who is in sole charge of them for so many hours out of the twenty-four; their behavior will be lax, or dignified and respectful, just according to her manner of deporting herself. Furthermore, she should never give away any of the provisions belonging to the ward. When a doctor is up very late with a patient, or is called several times during the night, he may feel the need of procuring something to eat, but the night-nurse of the ward is not the one to provide him with refreshment. In such matters the head-nurse is allowed some discretion, although it would be far preferable if the hospital provided other ways. Be that as it may, it is certain that a night-nurse's time is not at her own disposal for any such extra duties, neither is the food in the ward provided for any one except the patients. The nurse is caretaker not only of the occupants of her ward, but also of all that pertains to it and them.

In a private ward, where there may be more than one nurse, extra care should be taken that no noise or talking takes place. I should not emphasize this point, were it not for the fact that I have frequently known night-nurses, without any bad intention, but through pure heedlessness, to disturb patients by unnecessary noise and talking and entirely spoil their night's rest. Even a well person may find it no easy matter to get to sleep again if once awakened, and in the case of the sick it is usually even more difficult. Every night-nurse must know from experience how trying it is to be aroused by noise, when trying to get a much-needed rest during the day, and how hard it is to get to sleep again. A fellow-feeling, therefore, should make her remember to be very careful in this respect. In fact the golden rule, of doing to her patients as she would they should do unto her, must ever be in force.

A nurse should make frequent rounds among her patients throughout the night, for only by so doing will she be enabled to give a correct report as to how they have rested. A patient may be absolutely quiet all night and make no sign, although he may be getting but little sleep. Again, only in this way will it be possible for her to find out little wants or to add little comforts that she would otherwise miss. Just going to the ward door, and listening to see if all is quiet, is not enough. At the same time all her observations should be made so quietly that her presence will never disturb her patients. To be able to slip frequently into and out of the room, to note the condition and to take the pulse of a sleeping patient without awakening him, means the perfection of nursing. She should never forget, towards the early morning, to see that additional coverings are put over patients, who may feel the extra chilliness of those hours, and that hot cans are kept in readiness for anyone who needs them. All such attentions are included in true nursing; just the perfunctory carrying out of specified orders will not suffice. During my own training one of the first true lessons I ever received in nursing ethics came to me very forcibly upon hearing a patient say of the night-nurse, "Oh, Miss ____ is a good night-nurse, she takes such good care of her patients; if anyone of them wants a drink, she never brings it without first letting the water run until it is nice and cold, and she does everything in just that way."

There may be several nights, during a term of night-duty, when many of the beds are vacant, and there are few, if any, very ill patients to engross one's attention. At such times, especially if all the patients sleep fairly well, the hours of watching are apt to drag, and the desire to sleep becomes all but over-powering, unless the nurse finds occupation for her hands and mind. Her head-nurse usually anticipates such leisure time, by having some light work for her to do, in the way of mending, making some of the various kinds of pads and jackets, or copying charts. In a surgical ward this extra time is well spent in adding to the stock of bandages and surgical dressings, or in various other ways helping in keeping ahead with the necessary ward supplies. At the same time, all such work affords opportunities for practice. Novels, or books of any kind not connected with one's studies, should never be read on duty. In fact any kind of reading is apt to make one sleepy, and should not be indulged in, at least to any great extent, since it will often be hard enough to keep awake, even when extra inducements, such as reading, or sitting in too comfortable a rocking chair, are carefully avoided. For a sentinel to sleep at his post is a cardinal sin, that meets with extreme forms of punishment, and to sleep when on nursing duty is not a whit less culpable. A woman, who is untrustworthy enough to be guilty of so grave a misdemeanor, is not of the stuff of which nurses should be made and her services should be dispensed with at once. Keeping oneself occupied, and moving about, are the chief safeguards, whenever one is not busy with the patients, until the hour comes for the morning work to begin. Then, in any case, all desire for sleep vanishes; the patients are prepared for breakfast; the ward is given a general tidying up; the morning medicines are due; the bath-rooms and lavatories have to be left in good order and all utensils cleaned and put away. Finally, the night report has to be written up from regular notes made all through the night, which should be entered neatly and concisely in ink in the book set apart for this purpose. This report should deal, one by one, with the patients for whom special orders have been left, a clear but brief statement being made of what has been done for each. All new developments and the amount of nourishment taken should be carefully entered. No opinion should be expressed and nothing facetious attempted; a record of facts is all that is required. Convalescents, who are under no special treatment, and whose condition remains about the same night after night, do not require individual entries, but may be reported together. It must be remembered that night reports are official documents, to be placed on file, and that they may be produced at any time as evidence in a case. On this account, as well as for other obvious reasons, they should always be business-like and strictly true, with no added or diminished coloring on the part of the nurse. When finished, the report should be signed and handed to the head-nurse as she enters the ward. The night-nurse should remain until her head-nurse has read it, in order to make any further explanations or answer any questions, after which, all her other work being finished, she goes off duty and to her breakfast.

During their term of night-duty all the nurses are under the supervision of the head-night-nurse, both when on and when off duty. Although they receive their orders from their head-day-nurses and are responsible to them for executing them, it is the head night-nurse who makes visits at intervals, in order to judge how the orders are being carried out, and to supplement with her greater experience the inexperience of the pupil-nurse, so that it is necessary that she should be kept informed of everything that is going on in the ward. All the various orders and patients under special treatment should be talked over freely with her, so that she may make no mistakes in exercising her judgment, through not knowing sufficiently the details of any particular case. The responsibility she assumes is greater than that of her staff of night-nurses, and she looks to each one of them to assist her to meet it properly, by giving her a detailed account of all that is going on in the ward. On occasions when the work is heavy, or when in her judgment it is advisable to do so, the head-nurse may assist in taking care of the patients. This will afford the pupil a splendid opportunity for gaining information and experience, since she has all the advantages to be derived from private lessons both in practice and theory.

The need for the doctor's presence through the night is always determined by the head-nurse, except in grave emergencies, when the loss even of a few minutes' time might be of serious moment. In such cases the pupil-nurse must act on her own responsibility, but, generally speaking, her judgment is not sufficiently mature to enable her to make such decisions and she would probably often summon the physician unnecessarily. A nurse is never supposed to leave her ward under any pretext, since she can never know what may happen in her absence. Any extra supplies, help or messages, should be left for the head-nurse to arrange.

When off duty, the nurse is also responsible to the night head-nurse. Any absence from meals, change of hours, or remaining out of bed beyond the regular time, is only allowed in exceptional cases and must always be subject to her approval.

Night duty is also the time for the trial of a nurse's loyalty in regard to her school and her fellow-nurses. Until this time she may have been too strictly under observation, and too closely confined to her duties, to have had many opportunities for indiscretions in this way, but from now on she will come more generally into touch with her fellow-nurses, the physicians and other people. She will have many temptations and invitations to discuss her school affairs and those of the other nurses, but she must remember that, for the time being, she is a member of a large family and its privacy and internal affairs should be as loyally guarded as those of her own home circle. The individuality of each member of the family should be respected; the shortcomings or mishaps of any nurse should never be made a topic of conversation outside, either to friends in the city or to doctors. It is more than likely that nurses will meet with others, who are not specially congenial to them, or for whom they may have a positive aversion; but this fact affords no excuse for not showing absolute loyalty, or forever permitting any disparaging remarks to be made about another nurse, so long as she remains a member of the school. If she is unworthy of confidence and loyalty, one may be very sure that the fact will become evident sooner or later, inasmuch as such people, in the end, usually appear in their true characters. In the meantime, the principle of loyalty must be maintained, irrespective of personal feelings. Moreover, self-discipline in this matter will serve as a good training, preparatory to entering private families later on in her professional capacity, when the nurse will be expected to maintain strict silence on the subject of all family affairs.

Any tendency towards the formation of cliques in a school is to be discouraged; they are harmful to the best development of a true class spirit; are narrowing and apt to render unduly and unfairly critical those who are members of them. Sentimental, intense personal friendships between nurses are a mistake, and are rarely productive of good. In some instances they must be regarded as forms of perverted affection; they are always unhealthy, since they make too great demands upon the emotions and nerve force, and are likely to assume undue proportions, so as to interfere with the proper discharge of one's duties and with the habits necessary for good health and good work. A good steady, common-sense friendship will be more helpful to both parties and will assuredly last longer. Again, a nurse, who is deeply absorbed in one or more intense personal friendships, is less apt to appreciate and do her full share in maintaining the *esprit de corps* that must exist among all the members of the staff, in order that a high order of work may be maintained throughout the whole training school.

The first night-duty brings with it a reversal of the order of living, and amid the sudden change and the new responsibilities, it will sometimes be difficult for the young nurse to retain her usual mental equilibrium. I have gone somewhat into detail, because at such a time certain things — even friendships — are apt to assume undue proportions in the mind of the inexperienced pupil, and may thus lead to a warping of her judgment, just when the opportunities for a broadening out are becoming greater.

Chapter Nine - The Senior Nurse

The first half of the pupil's time, so far as the practical side is concerned, has usually been spent in receiving instruction in surgical and medical nursing, in the diet-kitchen, in assisting in the dispensary and emergency service, and in doing night duty, while along with her practical training there has been, it is to be hoped, a gradual development in the ethical side of nursing. Now, however, she takes rank as a senior nurse and all the time is being afforded increasing opportunities for meeting greater responsibilities. During this second period, her practical instruction will include a service in the operating-rooms, in the maternity ward, special duty with private patients, or with those who are critically ill, and ward administration. She will also be expected to acquaint herself more closely with her relations to the hospital as a whole, and its management in general, and I would add — what heretofore perhaps has not been generally taught — with her future duties and responsibilities towards her school alumnae. To the work of a senior nurse she is expected to bring special qualifications, as a result of her experience as a junior. By this time she should have lost any self-consciousness, that may have been noticeable and may have hampered her in the beginning, and should have attained to a certain quiet confidence and self-poise that will be needed in meeting her increased responsibilities. She will also be expected to exhibit a greater degree of skill and thoroughness than could justly have been demanded of her, before she had had time to acquire them by sufficiently long practice. Ranking as the first assistant of the head-nurse in the ward, not only will her usefulness be increased, but her influence and authority will be extended. Moreover, her future career as a graduate nurse will largely depend upon the degree of capability, which she shows in performing all the various senior duties. The success she achieves in the ward as a senior will largely determine her chances of becoming a head-nurse in the future. She may have ambitions in that direction, but she cannot expect her superintendent to encourage her in her desire and give her an appointment in her own school, or recommend her to any other, unless she has proved herself worthy of such a trust. Again, the probable measure of her future success as a nurse at large can be estimated pretty accurately by her manner of caring for her special patients; upon her work now, therefore, will depend whether she is recommended in unqualified tons of approval for private duty later on. Her absolute trustworthiness in matters of detail, in addition to her practical ability, will decide her fitness to take charge of an operating-room. For all these various reasons, therefore a senior should regard this latter part of her course as a period in which to perfect herself in practical nursing, as well as affording a good preparation for any administrative hospital duties, which she may desire to assume as a graduate nurse. Much still remains to be done; her time of probation has not yet passed; a foundation has been laid, but she must continue to build with unflagging zeal. Unfortunately, we sometimes find that, when a woman becomes a senior nurse, she relaxes somewhat in her efforts. This may be due partly to a reaction from the exertion put forth during the first portion of her training, or to a feeling that she already knows enough about her work to enable her to earn a living, and to a sense of security, owing to the lessened possibilities of dismissal. Whatever the reason may be, it is certain that any woman, who now exhibits signs of carelessness or of diminished zeal, has missed the true spirit of her work, and if she does not soon recover it, it would be better for herself as well as others, nurses as well as patients, that she should resign and find some other less responsible, less exacting work, and one requiring only a somewhat lower standard. A superintendent, therefore, watches with anxiety for proofs of real progress on the part of her seniors, for she recognizes the fact that evidences of having benefited by the first twelve or eighteen months' training must be clearly shown, and continued progress must be made, by all who are to be successful in their future work as graduates, and who will reflect credit upon the hospital, their school and their profession.

In the ward a senior nurse ranks second. It is, therefore, essential that the relation in which she stands to the head-nurse, who is her superior officer, and the rest of the staff, should be clearly defined and the limit of her authority understood, in order that nothing may interfere with the maintenance of that true harmony, which is necessary to the highest order of work. Constant misunderstanding or friction, distrust or suspicion, between the members of the nursing staff is soon apparent, and not only impairs the practical work, but also has a bad effect upon the patients, who are quick to feel and respond to the atmosphere among the nurses. The *esprit de corps* must be preserved at any cost to one's private feelings, and the senior nurse has it in her power to do double duty in this respect. She stands midway between the juniors, over whom she has a certain amount of delegated authority, and the head-nurse, who is in supreme command in the ward. As first assistant, and as acting head-nurse, when necessity requires it, she should at all times prove herself the right hand of her chiefs assisting her in instructing the younger nurses, and in observing how they do their work, in preserving discipline and harmony both among patients and nurses, in promoting order and system, and in watching the little details upon which the comfort and well-being of the patients so largely depend. She should be most careful, however, never to forget her subordinate position. She should do her part in a quiet, unobtrusive manner, and never give offence to those under her by assuming a too authoritative air. She should guard against over-officiousness and should take upon herself no unnecessary responsibility or authority, referring all doubtful questions to the head-nurse, when the latter is present. Tact and discretion will stand her in good stead in performing her duties as a senior nurse. She should give her head-nurse every reason to feel complete confidence in her, so far as her knowledge goes, everything she does being marked by such a degree of thoroughness and tactfulness, that the disagreeable necessity for criticizing the quality of her work, or putting her in her proper place, need never arise. She must gradually acquaint herself with all the details connected with the administration of the ward, in order that she may be capable of assuming that management when the head-nurse is off duty, or is called away for any reason, so that the work and care of the patients may go on undisturbed. A thorough knowledge of the patients and their treatment is necessary to enable her to reply intelligently to any questions the physicians may ask her about them, when she is left in charge. In a word, now is her opportunity to acquaint herself with a head-nurse's duties, if she hopes to take such a position herself in the future. The knowledge she can gain at this time will then be of the utmost value, as it will enable her to at once assume her new duties with ease and comfort to herself, her patients and all concerned, instead of sacrificing every one while she is gaining her experience. The successful performance of her administrative duties will demand good judgment and executive ability; without these the best of intentions will be productive of only sorry results. She is supreme in the ward only at such times as the head-nurse is absent. Hence, she should be discrete in the exercise of her authority. In her dealings with the probationers and juniors, she should always bear in mind that, not so very long ago, she was one herself and that she ought hardly to have had time to forget how she herself liked to be treated.

A senior's influence among the younger members of the staff is very often greater than she may be aware of, because she has in their eyes attained to a certain pinnacle of perfection and they look up to her accordingly. At the same time, since she is not so awe-inspiring a personage as a head-nurse, the pupil-nurses feel more at home with her and will be only too happy to listen to her instructions, provided she does not adopt too patronizing a manner and tone. She must also bear in mind that she has reached a stage in her training, when the results of her efforts in cultivating the ethical side of her work will have great weight with the juniors, and that what she does and what she says will encourage or discourage them in persevering and in doing what is right.

While it is always in order in a ward to detail a nurse of any rank to do work that may be regarded as more properly belonging to the probationer or junior, the senior nurse, generally speaking, does less of this part of the nursing, owing to the other demands upon her. Nevertheless, should the fortunes of war or some emergency throw such work in her way, she must guard against ever taking advantage of her position to put off on the younger nurses any rough, hard work which has been assigned to her, or imposing double duty upon them while she takes her ease. This would be taking mean advantage; the others will be quick to recognize such treatment and she will fall in their estimation accordingly. On the contrary, she may occasionally seize the opportunity of doing double duty, by assisting the juniors in work, which to them seems very hard, but which to her with her additional experience is quite easy.

Whenever a senior is left in charge she should be careful to note everything of any importance that has happened and upon going off duty, if her head-nurse be at home, she should make a careful report.

Throughout her course she is instructed by her head-nurse in the rules to be observed in her relations with the rest of the management of the hospital. Thus, for example, she learns what are the customs prevailing with regard to dealings with the housekeeping department, the kitchen, the laundry, the main business office and the superintendent of the hospital, in order that all may work in harmony and that no reflections may be cast upon the nursing department through her ignorance.

When detailed to special duty, that is, when the care of one patient is entrusted entirely to her, more especially if the patient belongs to the private ward, she will be afforded excellent opportunities for obtaining an insight into the exigencies of private nursing, as compared with those belonging to the regular hospital duties, and to a certain extent will also have an opportunity of proving the amount of tact at her command, when called upon to deal with patients in their own homes. In her first experience she must be very guarded in many directions. It is to be hoped she has not contracted that most objectionable habit of calling her patient a case; the word in itself has such a cold, hard, forbidding sound that I wonder nurses ever permit themselves the use of it, except when speaking in the abstract. Moreover, since patients themselves are apt to resent the term, it is just as well for a beginner to avoid its use from the start. On the other hand, a novice is liable to err in the opposite direction and to be too sympathetic, and is even in danger of becoming sentimental. A wise sympathy, tempered with judgment, is expected of every good nurse, but has no connection with the maudlin, too impulsive variety, which is an evidence of weakness. She will show her sympathy by thoughtful little deeds and acts far better than by many words, holding hands, or worse than all, by shedding tears. Whether as a special nurse or as one of the regular assistants in the private ward, she must not under any circumstances talk about one patient to another. To confide to another the disease from which one patient is suffering, whether he is likely to recover and the like, is a sin of which a nurse should never be guilty; to tell the names

of any new arrivals in the ward, to discuss the various visitors and their sayings and doings, would be equally reprehensible. In fact absolutely nothing
should be passed from one patient to another through the nurses. If a death
has occurred, it is not to be mentioned. Nor should the affairs of the institution, the officials, the physicians, or the other nurses, be made a source of
conversation or gossip. Patients and their friends soon recognize a nurse
who makes it a principle never to talk about such affairs, and although they
may be disappointed in not having their curiosity gratified, their respect for,
and confidence in, the nurse and the institution increases. An inquisitive patient once gave me it as her opinion that the nurses were "like so many
clams," for after being ten days in the hospital she had never been able to
find out, from one of them, who was her next-door neighbor, or what was the
matter with any of the patients. This was just as it should have been, and it is
only to be regretted that the complaint is not more often justified. With her
patients the nurse should be most reticent as to their true condition, if it is a
serious one. In some instances her position may be most trying. To the question often put to her, "Do you think I am going to get well?" she must, of
course, answer encouragingly, but with the utmost discretion, merely repeat-
ing what the physician has said in the presence of the patient. It is not her
part or privilege to express what she herself may think. She should never
allow herself to lose control of her emotions, and although she may feel bad-
ly, to the verge of tears, her sympathy must always take some other form.

When doing special duty in a private ward, the nurse is under the direction
and control of the ward head-nurse; in this respect she is in the same position as the other members of the staff; on coming on or going off duty she
reports to the head-nurse, to whom she also looks for the arrangement of her
hours. If she is on special night-duty and her time for rest comes in the morning, she should leave her patient and the room in perfect order before going
away, since she is usually relieved by the regular ward nurses and their time
is, of course, too much occupied in the morning to undertake the extra work.
A special nurse should leave all the dishes, instruments and various appliances she may have used, clean and in their proper places, just as she would
do in a private family. Any flowers should be well cared for, and little extra
delicacies, to be provided for her patient, should be her special care, so they
may surely be well prepared and that no mistakes may occur in this respect.

While going through her operating-room service, the nurse should be especially careful to train herself to be quick to observe, and to learn to anticipate what is wanted. Of course she should never offer anything before it is
asked for, but there is no harm in having it in readiness the moment it is
needed. This ability to keep ahead of the work, a keen observation and
promptness in action are always to be found in a good operating-room nurse.
Moreover, in these days of aseptic surgery, it is necessary to be strictly conscientious in every detail in the matter of cleanliness in preparing dressings,
solutions, instruments, and in fact in the care of everything which enters the

operating-room. Good or bad work here is often a matter of life or death to the patient, and only a strictly careful, observant woman, one that never slurs over the minutest details but who appreciates their value, ought to be entrusted with such a grave responsibility.

Bearing herself always with dignity, she should not neglect to demand at the hands of her staff the same degree of regard for the position they hold. The operating-room is no place for indulging in talking or frivolity of any kind, and during an operation strict silence should be maintained by the nurses, unless they are directly addressed.

Until this stage of her training, a nurse has had quite enough to do, if she has paid attention to the ethical subjects dealt with in the foregoing chapters, and has combined their development with growth in her practical studies. But in her senior year, the time begins to draw near when she will take her place in the outside world as a trained nurse. To be a worthy member of a profession implies certain obligations and duties, and in order to prepare herself to support these responsibilities she should, during the last months of her training, gladly avail herself of any means provided for this purpose. In connection with almost every school there is now to be found a flourishing alumnae, and in not a few schools special instruction is provided, in order to prepare pupils for the duties belonging to such associations. This special preparation will also enlighten the coming graduate as to what will be demanded of her as a member of a profession. The right to join her alumnae should be regarded as a distinct privilege, since it represents the one avenue through which she may keep in proper touch with her hospital and school, through which loyalty and devotion may be fostered, and through which she may the better learn to live for others and not just for her own small desires and by her own narrow views. Membership is also valuable as identifying her with her colleagues in good standing, since graduates are allowed to retain membership only so long as they bring no dishonor upon their profession. It is thus a safeguard in her professional life; and through it she will obtain an ever-increasing idea of the value of the practice of ethics in her career. Moreover, by utilizing the facilities afforded by the alumnae association, she will be enabled to keep up in her studies and remain in touch with any improved methods in nursing and with the changes in treatment in medicine and surgery. Above all, she must remember that only by the union of all nurses in one great body, through associations, can a standard be erected and maintained, that may become common to graduates from all good schools, and by which the best professional interests of nurses will be advanced. To understand one's personal obligations in all these respects requires time, thought and discussion; consequently, a senior nurse, who has not neglected these subjects during her training, will find herself prepared to at once assume her place as a graduate nurse, having a proper sense of her privileges and responsibilities and enough experience to become from the outset a valuable member of her profession.

Chapter Ten - The Head-Nurse

The work of a large training school attached to a modern hospital must necessarily be subdivided among several different departments, some of which have to do only indirectly with the patients. Naturally, the first and most important duty of the superintendent of the school is to supply proper care and nursing for the sick, and this by itself calls for a good deal of organization; but in addition, she is responsible for the training of her pupils, as well as for their physical, and to a certain extent also for their moral welfare. But in order that all these various duties may be properly performed, she must have helpers, and she therefore surrounds herself with a group of women, each of whom is assigned to a responsible position, and to whom the superintendent looks for assistance in carrying on both the nursing and the teaching work. From these assistants — each of whom has the title of head-nurse — one or more are selected to assist the superintendent in the work of general supervision; one is assigned to each hospital ward and operating room, one becomes head-night-nurse, another is made instructor in invalid feeding and is put in charge of the diet-kitchen, while still another is entrusted with the supervision of the Nurses' Home and sees that the comfort, health and general well-being of the nurses are not neglected. All these are positions of trust and responsibility, and each one in its own way, directly or indirectly, is of no mean importance in providing for the best interests of the sick, not only in the hospital itself, but also wherever its influence is carried.

The head-nurses, then, form a body, each member of which, in her own department, ranks next in responsibility and authority to the superintendent of the training school, and it is her duty to see that the department, of which she is put in charge, should be characterized by the highest degree of efficiency, while at the same time its work is carried on in harmony with that of the others, so that all together combine to supply the best nursing for the hospital and the best training for the pupil-nurses.

I know of no hospital appointment so attractive as the position of head-nurse in a large general hospital. It is true, it has its own peculiar hardships and worries — What work that is worthwhile has not these? — but it has also its great privileges, and the hardest burden of all — responsibility — need never be overwhelming, inasmuch as it is shared with the superintendent, who is responsible in the end, for the proper working of all the several departments.

In the arrangement and management of her ward and its every detail, the head-nurse has plenty of scope for the exercise of a goodly amount of executive ability; in her position as head of a department, she comes in direct contact with her patients, personally supervising all the various forms of treatment ordered by the physician, and thus can keep pace with the progress in nursing methods. Furthermore, although she is not expected to do much of the actual nursing herself, she is still able to keep herself in practice and in advance of her pupil-nurses, since part of her duty consists in teaching them the practical side of their work, while at the same time she has an incentive not to neglect her professional reading and studies. Again, in carrying on the work of her own department, she will of necessity often be brought into relation with that of others, so that she will have many opportunities of gaining a good practical insight into the general working of the different subdivisions and of the whole institution. As an official in the training school, which in many respects must be conducted on principles similar to those prevailing in other schools, the head-nurse has accorded to her a greater amount of personal freedom, than would be advisable in the case of the pupils, inasmuch as a riper experience and the acceptance of increased responsibility justly presume a lessened need of supervision. Thus, as was said before, the position of head-nurse is a desirable one for the right sort of woman, inasmuch as she can not only find a present happiness while busying herself with her duties, which are sufficiently varied to exclude any chance of monotony, but also at the same time can be continually broadening out, learning more and making herself more useful and more fitted for any other form of work she may assume later; nor need she ever fear that the years spent as head-nurse in a hospital will prove to be time wasted.

It has always seemed strange to me that the true value and importance of this position has never as yet been fully understood or appreciated by hospital authorities. The duties and responsibilities of a head-nurse are manifold, and come upon her from many sides. These relate to her own superintendent of the training school, the patients, the physician, the trustees of the hospital, represented by the superintendent, the heads of the different departments and the pupil-nurses. To meet successfully, and adjust oneself to the various conditions involved, is in itself no small task and requires an ability, education and tact beyond the common. The woman, who has once proved herself a successful head-nurse, has in her the ability to go further and become a successful superintendent, at least of a small institution. It follows, then, that the qualifications, that are considered essential for the latter to possess, in a modified degree, should be required of a candidate for the position of head-nurse. First and foremost, she must have good practical qualifications in the matter of an executive ability, such as can render system, order and thoroughness the rule of the day. A woman without any ideas of method should never be chosen as a leader of others; even although she may possess all the other virtues, she will inevitably demoralize everyone else who works with her. In order to command the respect and proper consideration of the medical staff, her nurses and the patients, she requires decision of character and forethought, tempered with good judgment and adaptability. In order to give the physicians absolute confidence that their patients will receive the best of care and attention from her, she requires skill in organization, so that all orders are executed promptly and literally. To fulfill her obligations to her pupil-nurses, who make up her staff of assistants, she must bring to her work not only a thorough knowledge of the principles of nursing, both in theory and practice, but also the ability to impart this knowledge. As a teacher, she must arrange that, instead of doing the work herself, her pupils shall learn to do it in the best possible way, so that they, in their turn, may become efficient and desirable nurses.

To the hospital authorities she must render a faithful stewardship, by always instituting a careful and economical administration of the supplies entrusted by them to her for the use of their patients, and by precept and by practice she should make her assistants feel that wilful extravagance is an unpardonable offence. To be worthy of her position and of so great a trust, she must have high ideals with regard to the carrying on of her work, and she should daily and hourly endeavor to put into practice her methods, in such a way as to stimulate those about her to do likewise. I am convinced that, if all the head-nurses in our hospitals were selected from women who, approximately at least, came up to such a standard, the results of their administration would very soon become apparent in the uniformly higher grade of nursing and nurses. Moreover, such a staff would also become the strong rallying point of the nursing department instead of one of its chief weaknesses, as it is today, for at the present time, in most hospitals in this country, the members of the staff of head-nurses by no means always represent those who during their course of training have made the best record for general efficiency, or who possess the special attainments suitable for such positions. It certainly would be desirable that such an appointment should be regarded as a special mark of distinction and honor but unfortunately, as matters stand at present, the selection has to be made from the best available candidates, many of whom could not command a higher salary elsewhere, although there are usually a few who, for some reason or other, are willing to do hospital work without regard to the remuneration. It is indeed fortunate that a certain number of thoroughly competent and self-sacrificing women are always to be found as head-nurses in hospitals, but this want of foresight on the part of hospital authorities inevitably results in the filling up of the remainder of the positions with women of second or third rate ability. Occasionally, parsimony is carried on to such a degree that, even in hospitals which have not the excuse of poverty, pupil-nurses are advanced, before the completion of their training, and are entrusted with the work and responsibility that should belong only to an experienced graduate. Such a procedure is manifestly unfair to the hospital, to the patients, and to the other members of the training school. The most desirable nurses — never very numerous — are naturally in demand outside the hospital, so that few are willing to remain on the nursing staff as head-nurses, because at the present day they are seldom offered a salary commensurate with that which they could command when engaged in other branches of nursing. Again, the usual custom is to select the head-nurses for the hospital from among the graduates of the school attached to it, vacancies being filled from the best of the last class graduated. While this system has its good points, from the fact that one naturally prefers to give the preference to one's own, and that it can also be utilized as a means for encouraging pupils to make their best efforts, and in holding their allegiance and their interest in the welfare of their own school and hospital, at the same time it not infrequently happens that, in a class of students recently graduated, there cannot be found a sufficient number possessing the proper qualifications to fill all the vacancies. In such a case, it would seem far better to pass over the non-efficient graduates and give the appointment to a nurse from some other school, who has already shown her fitness for such a position. Furthermore, these occasional selections from outside are often extremely beneficial, since an infusion of new* blood is likely to be followed by the introduction of new and desirable methods and changes, that are absolutely necessary, if the school is to be kept from falling into set ways and ruts, while at the same time it would have a healthy influence upon the pupils, in broadening their views and their attitude toward other schools. There is a growing demand for good head-nurses, and more is required from them than in former years. The increasing tendency in scientific medicine towards specialism must inevitably be accompanied by a need for more thoroughness and exactness in details, which must, as a rule, be left largely in the hands of the head-nurse and her assistants. Formerly, it was not uncommon to see medical and surgical patients occupying the same ward, and even now in some hospitals children, gynaecological patients, and those suffering from diseases of the skin, the eye, the ear, are still to to be found in the general surgical ward, while in the medical ward there may be an indiscriminate mingling of various kinds of diseases. Where such an arrangement exists, and where there is such a great mixture of work, the patients, as well as the head-nurse and her assistants, are at a serious disadvantage, inasmuch as proper systematic attention to details becomes almost an impossibility, where the demands are so numerous and diverge in so many directions; where one's attention is necessarily so divided, and where the orders of so many different physicians have to be carried out. In such a ward there is usually an unpleasant sense of hurry, bustle and confusion — an atmosphere very undesirable in which to train our pupil-nurses. Here there is great danger that system, order and thoroughness will be neglected, while the instruction of the pupils is apt to be given in a haphazard fashion. In hospitals where more recognition is given to specialism in medicine, since the division of the medical work is so arranged that the principal specialists have their own wards and assistants, there is naturally a more complete study of the details of any particular disease and its treatment, by which the nurse also profits, since she is required to be more systematic, exact and thorough in all the minutiae; and hence the habits so essential to good nursing are emphasized instead of being sacrificed. Moreover, the atmosphere of the ward is usually that of quiet and repose, of work being done well and on time, without undue haste or noise and without any over-tax on the strength of those whose duty it is to perform these arduous tasks. In this respect hospital authorities and physicians have still much to learn. They do not seem to appreciate the fact that where, as under the old system, the work in a single ward is so diversified, that their nurses are kept hurrying and scurrying pell-mell from one thing to another all through the day, without having time for proper thought or careful attention to details, they are being diligently trained in methods utterly opposed to the best principles of nursing. Is it fair that, after a nurse has graduated, the physician should turn round and arbitrarily demand from her qualities, which he has made it impossible for her to acquire during her training, — system, quiet, order, and a perfection of finish in the details of her work? Happily for nurses, the tendency nowadays is towards specialism, which naturally creates a greater demand for more head-nurses, of a superior quality, since the responsibilities and duties are steadily becoming greater and better appreciated.

The position held by a head-nurse is, therefore, in one sense just as important as is that of her superintendent, differing from it only in variety and breadth of the responsibility assumed. A superintendent's head-nurses should look upon themselves as her staff of officers, her right hand supporters and representatives, each one answerable to her for the thorough administration of her own particular department, subordinate only in the sense that in all good forms of government there must necessarily be one recognized head. The relations existing between a head-nurse and her superintendent should be those of absolute loyalty, faithfulness and confidence on both sides. Each head-nurse should consider it a privilege to be able to share the responsibility of her particular branch with her superintendent, and the utmost frankness should be maintained between them. I do not mean that every little detail in the matter of the ward administration need be discussed; on the contrary, the head-nurse should have perfect liberty, provided only that it does not interfere with the whole general plan or system, since it is clear that in essentials, or where fundamental principles may be involved, unity of effort necessitates a thorough understanding as to the main line of action to be pursued. Without a thorough knowledge of what is being done in the several departments, the superintendent would necessarily often act to some extent in the dark and the results would be defective, but with each head-nurse of her staff faithfully performing her part and keeping her superintendent in proper touch with her portion of the work, the administration as a whole is manifestly kept up to a certain standard and the results must be more satisfactory. Nor is it easy to over-estimate the influence exerted upon the pupils by the knowledge that the head-nurses and superintendent have this perfect understanding and are working as a single unit in the interests of all; they cannot fail to catch some of the same spirit, and in such a school there will be much less need for personal criticism, much less lack of loyalty and confidence, while there will be greater evidence of honor and integrity.

In order to obtain the best results, and in order that system, method and the best results in teaching and practice may be obtained, a head-nurse should manage her department as a part of the whole. No woman can be a law unto herself, in administering the affairs of her ward; if she tries to do her work without regard to that of the others, much confusion, repetition in teaching and general misunderstanding, must inevitably result. But to obtain a uniform system and method, it is necessary that there shall be a general understanding among all the various heads and their chief, and I know of no better way, by which this can be obtained, than by a system of conferences conducted by the superintendent, who should at such times give systematic instruction upon subjects dealing with the duties of head-nurses. One hour weekly will be sufficient for the explanation and discussion of plans and for the bringing forward of new methods. Each head-nurse should keep a little note-book, in which any ideas, which may strike her, can be entered, so that, at the weekly meeting, questions of general interest may be asked, experiences that may help the others may be related, and any new and better methods in nursing may be brought forward and discussed. The progress of the various pupil-nurses may be considered; the needs of individuals who, in the judgment of their head-nurses, have been found to require extra attention or consideration, may be discussed and provided for; difficulties may be talked over and cleared up, and plans of action decided upon. Of course, each head-nurse will at times feel the need of talking over her ward affairs privately with the superintendent, since the general conferences will take up only such subjects as are of general interest to all.

It is obvious that all departments cannot be run exactly alike, but the broad lines may be the same. In all there will be the same general division into junior, intermediate and senior work, the same systematic way of teaching, the same length of time to be devoted by a pupil to each branch of work in the ward, as for instance, the care of the medicine closet, the giving of medicines, the taking of pulses and temperatures, charting, the care, preparation and serving of nourishment. A record system for each pupil should be kept by her head-nurse, so that upon leaving the ward to go to another she carries with her an exact statement of the branches of work in which she has had full or partial training, during her stay in that ward, and also of any in which she has been found deficient. Provided with this information, the next head-nurse may start from where the teaching and practice were left off and thus avoid repetition, as well as give the pupil the chance of making up her deficiencies, by allowing her to devote time to those branches in which she has had little or no experience. The mere fact that a pupil has spent a certain time in any given ward does not, by any means, imply that she has learned all there is to be learnt there, and the deficiencies, when she leaves one department, can to a large extent be remedied in others. System in teaching is all important, and unless the head-nurses agree upon the same broad outlines, the ground can never be thoroughly covered. Each head of a department should make out a scheme of what can be done for her pupils while under her care, both as regards practical work and also the amount of theory she thinks necessary to employ, in order to make everything clear. With this as a starting point, she should try and arrange the time of each nurse and her own duties, in such a way that each practical subject, in whatever branch of nursing the pupil may be employed, may be gone over carefully. In addition to this regular teaching, she should always make it a point to allow her whole staff the privilege and benefit of hearing about or seeing any unusual form of disease, or treatment, that may arise, and that her pupils might not have an opportunity of encountering again in their course of training.

But side by side with her instruction in the theory and practice of nursing, she must ever bear in mind that it is her duty to inculcate and enforce the ethical principles, appreciating the fact that no one other person has the same opportunity as the head-nurse in this respect. She should be keenly alert to each pupil's failings or successes in this regard, and she should insist, by precept and example, that the laws of ethics, written and unwritten, should be strictly observed. Her attitude towards all of her nurses should be one of the utmost impartiality. Not the shadow of favoritism should exist, nor should there ever be anything in the way of warm personal friendships between the head-nurse and her pupils. If such exist, the best interests of the patients must sooner or later suffer, for it is rarely possible for the chief to criticize the work of an assistant, who is her intimate friend, or to make her do it over and over again, without creating dissatisfaction. The head-nurse must either sacrifice her self-respect and fail in the proper performance of her duty, or lose her friend, and in either case unhappy results must ensue. Moreover, evidences of partiality are at once perceived, and silently or openly protested against by the other pupils, with the result that the harmony of the whole department is destroyed. Each pupil requires, for her own good and advancement, a certain amount of judiciously administered censure, praise or encouragement, as occasion demands, although the manner of giving it must be regarded. To reprove a pupil with any show of impatience, or in the presence of patients or other nurses, is likely to result in more harm than good. It is much better to quietly suggest that the work must be repeated, until it is finished in a satisfactory manner, and at the same time to make her understand that it must be done better in future. If these kindly methods are not successful, after repeated efforts, or if the pupil is beyond the management of her head-nurse, the matter should be referred to the superintendent of the school, to be dealt with after due consideration of all its various aspects. Such a method of procedure, of course, applies only to cases in which a pupil has failed to do satisfactory work from pure ignorance or inexperience. Where neglect or bad care of the patient has been wilful, the reproof should be direct and, if necessary, should be given in the presence of the patient, in order that the sick may understand they have redress for all just grievances. The bestowal of praise also needs a good deal of judgment.

Injudicious commendation is apt to make the receiver conceited, while others, who are trying hard to do their best, are discouraged, because they are passed over. Furthermore, it is better to train nurses to work not for praise — which later on they may not receive even when they have rightly deserved it — but rather because to render good honest service is right at all times and under all circumstances.

In her official reports to her superintendent on the character of the work done by her pupils, and the ability shown by them, the head-nurse should always take care to show no partiality, and her decisions should be arrived at only after much thought and careful observation.

But while the head-nurse endeavors to be just and kind in her dealings with her pupils, it is her duty to exact from all implicit obedience, punctuality, thoroughness and a hearty co-operation in all that pertains to the life of the ward. Her own personal dignity need never be of a nature to make her unapproachable by her pupils or to inspire them with fear or dislike. A disinterested single-heartedness of purpose in her work, and in her dealings with them, will help her to succeed better and command more respect than a frigid aloofness, which would show that her dignity is of the kind that must always be on guard and needs to be carefully sustained.

The careful instruction and oversight of her nurses are intimately associated with good care for the patients, who must ever hold the first place in her thoughts. In her relations with them, the head-nurse is the responsible representative of others. She undertakes that the physician's wishes in regard to their treatment are carried out, while at the same time she is entrusted by the hospital authorities with the duty of seeing that everything, that is provided for the comfort and well-being of the patients, is put to the best use. She is the person upon whom the patients chiefly depend; they look to her for the proper attention, and appeal to her, when they think they are being neglected. It is through her planning and influence that they are surrounded with a pleasant atmosphere and the best of care; the actual manual labor must, in the main, be in the hands of her assistants, but the head-nurse must ever be on the alert to see how both patient and nurse are faring. Her treatment of them must be impartial, considerate and always kindly, and she should insist that each one on her staff does likewise. A head-nurse cannot be too vigilant in seeing that the patients are receiving proper care and attention, for she can judge, better than any one else, if they are happy and satisfied with their nursing and treatment, or the reverse. She must remember that upon her, to a great extent, depends the making or marring of the reputation of the hospital. It does not do to trust too much or to leave too much to the discretion of her assistants; her own personal supervision is indispensable. She should see that everything is in readiness for the regular daily visits of the medical staff to their patients, that the ward is quiet and orderly, that the patients and beds are presentable, and that she herself and her staff are ready to accompany the physician. She should always have her senior and one other nurse at least attend her at rounds; the senior stays by her side to help when necessary, while the junior brings anything that may be required, or assists in various other ways. Both the head-nurse and her senior should be familiar with the treatment ordered for each patient and able to answer, readily and clearly, any questions that may be asked; no one but the head-nurse, however, is expected to reply, unless she is directly appealed to by the latter. She should have her assistants trained to be on the alert to anticipate her wishes for anything needed, so that few words, if any, will be necessary during rounds. The various books for records should be carried and all orders promptly entered, at the time they are given, so as to insure that nothing shall be forgotten. Rounds should be conducted in a dignified, professional manner, befitting the gravity of the work in hand. Unnecessary conversation should not be indulged in, nor should the least trace of levity be countenanced. Although a quiet cheerfulness has a good effect upon the patients, any semblance of jesting is not only undignified, but is out of place in the presence of sickness and suffering. The head-nurse herself should set a good example in this respect, and should never speak, unless in direct answer to the questions of the physician.

The daily rounds also afford an opportunity for training the pupils in the proper deportment and etiquette to be observed towards physicians, in the hospital or in private families. The head-nurse and her staff should stand to receive the visiting physician, and from the moment of his entrance until his departure, the attending nurses should show themselves alert, attentive, courteous, like soldiers on duty; there must be no lounging up against beds or chairs, no signs of indifference or carelessness. Such breaches of etiquette are unpardonable, although I recall with regret instances, in which a nurse on private duty, who had been trained to do better, has committed just such errors, and even worse, and has then felt aggrieved, because she was sharply criticized for such behavior.

To all the various hospital officials her demeanor should always show a quiet courtesy. Whenever the superintendent of the hospital makes his tour of inspection, she should always be ready to show him everything in and about the ward, that he may be able to judge for himself that her care of the hospital property is what it should be. She should co-operate with him in managing, judiciously and economically, the outlay of hospital funds, by giving careful heed to what and how much she orders, and to the proper dispensing of supplies. In the matter of ordering food, linen, medicines, and other necessaries, as well as in their use, she should strive to attain a happy mean between extravagance and parsimony, for the daily saving in these items alone, in the aggregate, largely affects the total expenditure. In these matters, also, it is her bounden duty to teach her pupils the exercise of proper management and economy. In order to do the best work, it is not necessary for her to have a superabundance of supplies; a sufficiency, used intelligently, will serve the same purpose and mark the well-trained nurse. It should be her pride, as well as her pleasure, to help to build up and make stronger the institution, of which the training school is an integral part, for in the end the latter will reap its share of the increased usefulness of the hospital.

The influence of the head-nurse in the school proper, when added to that of the superintendent, can go far towards promoting a healthy tone in the community, as well as in maintaining discipline and good order in the nurses' home. If placed at the head of a table full of juniors, in a quiet way — and more by example than by precept — she can do much to encourage a good form of conversation, good table manners and uniform courtesy.

So important and useful a member of the family and hospital is the head-nurse, that many demands are likely to be made upon her, and in her unselfish interest and enthusiasm, she is liable to do too much and not give the necessary thought and care to her own health, unless her superintendent in turn keeps a watchful eye upon her and occasionally exercises a kindly interference. For the sake of her own health, as well as to emphasize her own teachings it is necessary that she shall be as punctual in observing the hours allotted her for duty as any of her pupils. During working hours she should give herself up to what she has on hand, in full unstinted measure; nor should she forget that in her case, also, there may be a danger of mere eye-service, unless, she is most conscientious. There is surely something wrong, somewhere, when a head-nurse needs to spend hours sitting over her books and lists, but can find leisure to talk to the doctors, for a half hour or an hour at a time, and when she never attempts to do any practical work with her own hands, even in the way of teaching. Nor is it her privilege, when on duty, to leave her ward to visit any other head-nurse. The times should be rare when she is not found in her place; and when for any reason she is obliged to be absent, even for five minutes, she should leave her senior in charge. Her patients should never be left entirely alone and a ward should never for a moment be without a recognized head. But when she has given good faithful service, while on duty, she should make it a point to leave her ward punctually, and for the time being, to put the cares belonging to it behind her, turn her mind to other things and seek some proper physical and mental recreation. Occasionally, for instance on Sunday mornings or some special holiday, it is well to leave the ward in the entire charge of the senior nurse and the pupils. By so doing, it will be possible for the head-nurse to form an accurate estimate of her own methods of training and of the ability of her pupils, for only a well-equipped ward will stand the test successfully; moreover, as a result of the added confidence placed in them, the nurses are apt to do better even than when their chief is present.

In conclusion, then, I would repeat that the position of a head-nurse, although trying in many ways, is one, above all others, in which an unselfish, capable woman has the largest opportunities for doing good work in a variety of ways. The full ability to meet her large responsibilities will not come to her in a day or a week; it must be the outcome of much endurance and perseverance, combined with well-directed energy and intelligence.

Chapter Eleven - The Graduate Nurse - Private Duty

At the present day when a pupil nurse has finished her course of instruction and has graduated, she has the good fortune to find a variety of work ready at hand, from which it is possible for her to select the career which is best adapted to her tastes, disposition and ability. Thus she has open to her positions which will enable her to continue her hospital work, district nursing and several kinds of private nursing, work in a physician's office, or the charge of the infirmary in a school or college — all interesting and attractive in their several ways. And although it is of advantage to her to spend a certain amount of time in broadening herself by gaining a practical experience in several of these branches, it is always best to select ultimately some particular line of work which she then should regard as her real profession, upon which she must bestow the best of her time, energy and talents. Furthermore, having chosen, she should at once set about making herself especially proficient in this particular branch, so that she may be sure to follow the best known methods, or may possibly, as her experience becomes more mature, work out new ideas of her own. The great mistake that a newly graduated nurse is apt to make lies in thinking that, having just completed a two or three years' training in nursing, she is fully equipped and knows all that is necessary to know on the subject. Curiously enough this is particularly true in regard to private nursing, whereas, as a matter of fact, this branch represents the rock upon which so many go to pieces and is the one in which we encounter the largest percentage of partial or absolute failures. I have more than once heard it stated that the hospital training-schools do not properly equip their pupils for the duties and exigencies of private nursing. But although this may be true to a certain extent, it would seem that the main cause of the failures, which we see, are due not so much to the training-school as to the graduates themselves. All that the former can possibly do is to carefully teach the pupil the theory and practice of nursing, while at the same time it surrounds her with an atmosphere which should give her a due appreciation of the responsibilities she is undertaking; the broader knowledge and experience, the recognition of the proper manner in which to act under new surroundings, which are not to be found in hospitals, can only be gained in time and by the exercise of much diligence. Just as in the case of the physician or lawyer, the success or failure of the graduate nurse will always depend only partly upon the school in which she has studied, but mainly upon her own efforts and upon her capacity for adapting herself to the work which she has undertaken.

In saying this, I would by no means be understood as holding the view that the principles of nursing that hold good in the hospital are not in the main applicable elsewhere, although it would seem as if some graduate nurses did their very best to forget what has been taught them and sometimes to act in direct opposition to these teachings. Private duty is the branch of nursing which absorbs the greater number of our graduates and it is to be feared that the majority rush into it without giving the matter any special consideration. Before undertaking a hospital position or beginning district nursing, or any other less usual form of work, the graduate, as a rule, goes through many searchings of heart before she decides that she has sufficient ability to justify her in attempting them; but for private duty all women seem to think themselves equally well qualified without further thought or effort. Is it to be wondered at that in many cases the result is total failure or at best only a small measure of success?

Private duty calls for its own special equipment and its peculiar qualifications. So far as the broad principle of one's work and the spirit in which it must be done are concerned, they are always the same, no matter where the field lies, but in private duty the nurse will encounter many conditions, which in the nature of things do not exist in hospitals, and which will necessitate certain modifications in the methods to which she has been accustomed. For the acquirement of the necessary knowledge it is impossible to lay down specific rules which will be applicable to every new emergency. Much must be left to experience — the only thorough teacher — and to the tact and adaptability of the individual. Nevertheless, it is to be hoped that lessons derived mainly from the failures of those who have gone before may go a certain way in helping the beginner to avoid some of the more common pitfalls, and in saving her from a few at least of the mortifications which will otherwise inevitably fall to her lot in the early part of her new career.

In undertaking the care of her first patient outside the hospital the young graduate will at once begin to understand that she is now working under different conditions. At the very outset the reception accorded her by the family may be a source of discouragement to her, although later on she may be willing to confess to herself that some of the disagreeable features have been due to her own inexperience in initiating professional relations with strangers. In assuming her duties, she will perhaps realize first of all that for hours at a time she is thrown entirely upon her own resources and must meet responsibility unaided; that between the visits of the physician she has only her own judgment to rely upon; that in sudden emergencies she Cannot now lean on others, but others will lean on her. In the hospital her work was mapped out for her. Her duties included certain services to be rendered to a set number of patients and a regular share of the ward work. Now, on the contrary, she finds that her whole time is to be devoted to a single patient; her various duties are not specifically pointed out to her, and she is left to her own resources in the organization of her work. Even if she has from time to time, while in the hospital, been entrusted with the charge of a special patient in one of the private wards, so that she has some idea of what this individual care means, she will find that certain modifications of her hospital methods are necessary, and the question how she can spend her whole time profitably upon one patient will be somewhat of a problem.

One of the first difficulties that she often encounters is one which is new to her and comes as a sort of surprise. Anyone with any experience in these matters knows that in a hospital an atmosphere prevails which seems to render the patients more amenable to treatment, especially from a mental standpoint. But the same patient who in a hospital would be most tractable and would rarely make any fuss about the carrying out of the physician's orders, when at home, and surrounded by over-sympathetic relatives and friends, will often prove refractory. In such cases the greatest tact will often be necessary in order to overcome whims and caprices, which run counter, to his best interests, and in order that the physician's orders may be strictly carried out without antagonizing either the sufferer or the members of his household. First of all, then, unbounded tact and patience are necessary, and in the beginning it will usually be found that the main problem to be solved is very largely how best to adapt herself to the new surroundings. The real nursing work, however, must be carried out in very much the same way in one place as in another, although the ever shifting and changing accessories may at times be somewhat bewildering. Whereas in the hospital her hours for work, meals and rest, were fixed, now she finds them uncertain and variable. Sometimes, in cases of serious illness and when no capable person can be found to relieve her, her hours on duty are long, and she can get but little rest and little if any recreation. Furthermore, she has many and various demands made upon her from many different sides, from which she was free in her hospital work. Then she knew to whom she was responsible — to her patient, the physician, and her superintendent. As it is now, the physician, the patient, the family, the friends and her profession, have all to be considered. In a well-organized hospital, where so many patients have to be cared for, as a matter of economy of time and energy, all that a nurse needs in her work is kept ready to hand. But in a private family it may be very different. Here, in most cases she will find little or nothing in the way of conveniences, except perhaps some few that she may have brought with her. But this is no great hardship if she has ingenuity enough to enable her to make the most of the materials at her command. Nor should she be too punctilious or too ready to think that she is being imposed upon. In sudden emergencies, or in cases of critical sickness, the relatives and friends are often so unnerved and helpless, that the nurse may see that some work, that would ordinarily be quite outside her duties, ought to be done and yet there is no one to be found at the time being who is capable of doing it. On such occasions let her not fear that she will compromise her dignity by doing what is necessary; when the emergency is over a nurse with tact can readily arrange matters so that no one in the household will think of asking her to do work other than that she has engaged to do.

Again, there are many uncertainties and many ups and downs in the life of a Woman who undertakes the nursing of the sick in private families. Sometimes she will meet with absolute hardships — bad lodging and bad food, and worse than all a capricious and ungrateful patient and fault-finding relatives — while at other times she will find herself surrounded by every luxury and made much of by the patient and her friends. It may be hard to find no separate room, an uncomfortable bed, or merely a sofa, nowhere to bathe, dress, eat, and sleep except in the patient's room; but such circumstances are fraught with less danger to the disposition and character of the nurse than an atmosphere of affluence and adulation. Let her look well to it that she finds herself ready to meet not only hardships but also these more subtle pit-falls, by steadily seeking to acquire during her years of training a philosophy that considers as essentials not the externals of life, but the satisfaction that comes from a sense of duty done. Then, and then only, will she not be deterred by hardships, or made too unhappy by neglect and thoughtlessness, nor spoiled by too much ease and injudicious praise. Again, it is not always easy for her to accustom herself to strange doctors, who may be quite' unlike those she has met with in the hospital; and whose methods may be different. In this connection it is all-important for her to remember that her responsibility ends when she has faithfully carried out the directions of the attending physician, and that obedience and loyalty to him are required of her. Her behavior towards other nurses, whether they be old fellow-pupils or come from some other training school, must always be characterized by the utmost fairness and tact so that all friction may be avoided. When two nurses who are associated together in the care of a patient cannot get on together, or when the slightest suspicion of rivalry or jealousy exists between them, good work cannot be done; moreover, the patient and the members of the family are quick to perceive any disagreement, and the reputation of the profession at large suffers on account of the pettiness of individual members.

The period of convalescence and the care of a case of contagious disease, in which the nurse is isolated from her fellow-creatures for weeks or months, make large demands upon her patience and upon her resources, both as regards the welfare of her patient and of her own mental and physical health. At such times the tediousness and the loneliness will often be unbearable, unless the nurse has learned the lesson of self-discipline and feels that the work is there for her to carry out to the end, for any weariness in well-doing will vitiate what has already been accomplished.

Enough has been said to show that in choosing private nursing a woman undertakes many responsibilities and anxieties from which hospital work is comparatively free. Much more could be added, but these pages are written with the hope of instructing, and in no way with the intention of deterring any honest, capable woman from taking up this important branch of our work. Let anyone who may feel somewhat discouraged, and who may think that impossibilities are demanded of her, remember that difficulties do not all come at once, and that often, for many cases in succession, none but the most pleasant experiences may be encountered. On the other hand, whereas it is of comparatively little credit to a nurse in a hospital to make everything go smoothly, even in the best ordered private houses difficulties and trials are always likely to be met with, so that the greater honor rests with the woman who makes a notable success in private duty. But whenever unpleasant or arduous duties or moments of anxiety are her lot, the nurse should regard them as so many opportunities for developing and strengthening her self-reliance, self-control, endurance, unselfishness and tact. Even the most trying circumstances need not daunt her, for she has only to remember that the long lane that has no turning does not exist in her work, but that, as a rule, it is a question of a few days, weeks, or at the most of months, after which she will be free to go on her own way again. The certainty that a change for the better is soon coming will enable her to meet trying situations cheerfully and patiently, and patience and cheerfulness go far towards ensuring success.

Private duty has its bright side and attractions to offset the disagreeable part. Many nurses prefer it because of their comparative freedom when disengaged, since the discipline and routine that must necessarily exist in hospital work after a time become somewhat irksome. The remuneration is also a matter of great importance to many, especially to those who have others dependent upon them, since the successful nurse is likely to be kept busy ail the time she desires and commands a good income. The various new experiences met with all help to broaden her knowledge of her work, of people, places and things, and to develop and strengthen her character. Moreover, the fact that her influence and usefulness may be greater for good than in almost any other work in which women are occupied in itself makes the life attractive, while there must always be a certain pleasure in overcoming unexpected difficulties, or obstacles that may seem all but insurmountable. Above all, it is a distinct pleasure and privilege to enter a family, which is distraught with fear over the illness of a loved one, and to pour oil on the troubled waters and to share with the physician the work of relieving suffering, of restoring health, saving life and preventing disease — motives which should be mainly responsible for her choice of nursing as a profession.

A graduate, therefore, who thinks of selecting private duty for her special branch of nursing, should consider carefully in how far she is fitted to meet the responsibilities connected with it, and what special qualifications she can bring to it. Moreover, she should try to clearly define in her own mind what her relations to her patient, the family, friends and the physician should be, as well as to determine the scope of her duties and responsibilities towards the public and her profession. Her attitude of mind towards her work will influence the performance of all her duties and will reveal itself to others at every turn. From the very start she must have ideals, and to these she must hold fast through good and evil report and through all kinds of ups and downs. We do not set up for ourselves ideals with the expectation of ever fully realizing them in this world, but if we do not keep before us a certain standard of perfection as a goal at which to aim, we more easily lose sight of many of the higher and better possibilities that lie in almost anything we may undertake. High thinking will go far to aid the nurse in forming good professional habits, which cannot fail to render the most difficult work not only easy but pleasant. But once having settled upon her ideals she should start from the first in a practical straightforward way which will render them every day more and more real to her. Her work has been undertaken as a voluntary act; she has not been forced to engage in it; let her then give herself up to it fully and freely with an undivided, cheerful heart. Even honesty of purpose and the desire to give full weight and measure and to do all things with all one's might bear better fruits when an immediate reward is found in the enjoyment of the work itself.

But in starting out to do private nursing, even before she takes charge of her first patient, it is advisable for the nurse to consider carefully certain minor questions on subjects connected with this particular branch. In the first place she has to supply herself with a certain number of uniforms, and certain appliances, which she will always need to have with her. At the same time she can decide in a general way as to her arrangements for taking care of her own health, the time she expects to devote to recreation and study, and whether she wishes to limit herself to the cafe of certain diseases.

An element of business must necessarily enter into the making of professional engagements, but this should not be carried too far, or prevent suitable modifications to meet particular cases. Engagements to nurse a patient may be made in several ways-; sometimes they come directly through the physician; at other times through the directory for nurses. Not infrequently a message is received directing a nurse to go to a given address, with perhaps only a meagre or no explanation as to the condition of things she may expect to find there. Later on, as a nurse becomes better known, the call often comes through some member of the patient's family. Occasionally the patient herself may wish to see the nurse before she definitely engages her services to take care of her after an operation or during the puerperium. At such an interview the attitude of the nurse should never be too stiff or too rigidly professional; her manner should be pleasant, so that the patient, who may have a dread of what is coming upon her, can feel that she will have someone with her on whom she may rely to be a comfort to her, morally as well as physically. Nor should the nurse assume a dictatorial manner or show any disposition to unduly insist upon her rights and privileges or the arrangements for her own comfort. Upon one point, however, both sides cannot be too business-like. There must be a definite understanding as to the exact date at which the engagement is to begin; and no matter how often patients or their families may fail in this respect, let it never be said of a nurse that she has been guilty of breaking an engagement wilfully or without just cause. She must always be one who, having sworn to her neighbor, disappointeth him not though it be to her own hindrance. To break such an obligation lightly, or to be unpunctual in meeting it, should be regarded as an unpardonable offence. It may happen that as soon as one has' made an engagement, another will be offered, which promises a higher remuneration, less work and more pleasant surroundings. At the very outset of her career let the nurse determine that her word shall always be kept, and that she will never yield to such a temptation. As a matter of fact, also, in this as well as in other matters, honesty will in the long run prove to be the best policy, for patients, physicians, or superintendents of training schools, who are often asked to recommend nurses, are not likely to forget dishonorable conduct of this kind.

Again, when a nurse, by putting down her name in the directory, has once signified that she is ready to take charge of a patient, she virtually engages from that time on to hold herself in readiness to respond to a call at a moment's notice. She should take no chances, on the possibility that she will not be wanted, and go off to spend the day in the country or to do a long morning's shopping. Even when she goes out for a short walk, she should always leave specific directions with some reliable person as to her whereabouts and as to the length of time during which she will be absent. Only those who have had charge of a nurses' directory know how unbusiness-like, careless and even dishonest, nurses can be in this respect, and how slow they are in understanding that the entering of their names in the register morally binds them to keep within call. I am well aware that such wrong-doing is rarely intentional and that dishonesty as applied to it seems a hard word, since it usually results from mere carelessness and thoughtlessness — faults, however, which are inexcusable in nurses, and are not compatible with a training which renders one worthy to deal with such grave responsibilities as life and death. Strict punctuality and an absolute living up to agreements are even more necessary in the case of a woman engaged in private nursing than when she was in the hospital. A nurse, not only to be successful but also to be honorable, must make for herself a reputation for never being late at an appointment, for always being on hand at a moment's notice to take a patient, when once registered, and for never breaking an engagement to go to a patient.

A nurse should never leave a patient on account of her own private affairs or because her position has been rendered disagreeable to her by the friends, the physician or the patient herself, unless she is assured that her presence will be productive of harm to the patient. But whenever circumstances have rendered her departure absolutely necessary, the nurse should do her utmost in helping to obtain a competent substitute and should be willing to remain until one can be found. Unless she is seriously ill herself, I can imagine no circumstances under which a nurse would be justified in leaving a patient until her place is filled. Even in cases in which her self-respect is clearly involved, it cannot be compromised by a strict adherence to duty, which consists in seeing that the patient shall not be sacrificed.

A good deal might be said about the 'duty of nurses as regards contagious diseases. In the past, I fear that this has not been clearly understood, and I can call to mind not a few instances in which members of the profession have repeatedly refused to take care of such patients. The existence of this attitude among so many nurses is one of the strong evidences of the absence of an accepted code of ethics and a consequent lack of a proper comprehension of their moral duties as members of a profession. One hears sometimes of physicians who have spent valuable hours in vainly trying to find a disengaged nurse who was willing to take a case of scarlet fever or diphtheria, and yet have met with a firm refusal at every turn. Is it to be wondered at that those who have had such an experience — though perhaps only once or twice — should deny that nurses, as members of a profession, have any ethical code, and that they promptly cross off -their list of desirable nurses the names of all the women who have refused, no matter how competent they may previously have shown themselves. This I know personally to have been the case in several instances, and in different cities, and to judge from the experience of other superintendents and of physicians, this condition of affairs would seem to be too general.

There are many reasons given by nurses why they will not take care of patients suffering from contagious diseases, but investigation will hardly justify many of them. If a nurse undertakes to do general nursing it is her bounden duty, no less than that of the physician, to take whatever case may come to her. Except on substantial grounds, she should never refuse a call to a sick person and she should never allow her personal inclination, her personal pleasure, or her personal gain to prevent her from going. As in the case of the physician, she must aid the suffering when called upon, without sitting down first to count the cost; nor has she the moral right to pick and choose her patients. If, however, she has selected a certain branch of nursing as her specialty, and is known not to take other cases, under ordinary circumstances she would be justified in refusing, although in an emergency, or when she is the only available nurse and the case is extreme, the claims of humanity might decide her to accept. Furthermore, if she has a definite engagement to take charge of an obstetrical or a surgical patient in the near future, it would not be allowable for her to nurse a case of contagious disease.

It is hardly necessary to say that all good reasons for a refusal, as soon as they were mentioned to a physician, would be readily appreciated. On the other hand, if a nurse declines to go through fear of her own personal safety, there is no excuse for her. She should have settled that question before she ever entered a hospital, for she must have known that there she would be expected to take any case assigned to her, and that any day she might be exposed to risks of various kinds. Such a position is very much on a par with that of a man who has enlisted as a soldier and then later on wishes to make the proviso that he shall always have the privilege of fighting in the rear, well protected against any chance of being shot. Moreover, now that bacteriology has cleared up so much for us as to the nature of infectious and contagious diseases, and when nurses are taught the best methods of avoiding infection, there is still less excuse for such conduct. Nowadays when nurses have contracted an infectious disease through simply caring for such patients, one is justified in saying that, in the majority of cases, such a misfortune has been due to some carelessness in dealing with their patients or to ignorance of the prophylactic measures, this employment of which would at least have minimized the risk. Fearlessness with regard to personal danger, coupled with an intelligent cautiousness when nursing any form of infection, will prove a nurse's best safeguards, and in the majority of cases will bring her through the ordeal unscathed, whereas, if she shrinks from the danger, she loses the esteem of her co-workers as well as of the physician, and, worse still, her own self-respect. But while a certain lack of personal courage might possibly be regarded as a weakness, more to be pitied than blamed, the same leniency is out of place where other ignoble reasons for shirking a plain duty are concerned. To refuse to go to the help of a sufferer because one dislikes the isolation that must necessarily be encountered; because one must submit for a time to be shut out from the rest of the worlds without liberty to meet one's friends, being obliged to take even one's recreation in solitude, does not enter the mind of the true nurse. To be deprived of the privilege of getting one's patient off one's mind for an hour or so in the day and of seeking mental refreshment among other surroundings — meeting a friend for a little chat, or going to one's own home if only for an hour — may be hard to bear, especially when the isolation lasts for weeks. But if the outlook is not agreeable, and the reality is still worse, are we ever justified in putting self before a duty which we have voluntarily engaged ourselves to perform? Again, where self-respect is involved, shall we be deterred from doing our duty by any pecuniary consideration? So far as money is concerned, the nurse may lose more than she gains by taking charge of a patient suffering from an infectious disease, inasmuch as, after leaving him, she is bound to avoid any risks of carrying the infection, and for this reason she has to remain idle a certain number of working days, during which she must pay for her own support. Again, this time is often unnecessarily prolonged, since it is often hard to satisfy a family, or even the physician, that the danger is past, so that her financial loss may be considerable. But such considerations should be allowed to have no weight when duty calls her to take her share of what comes, and in the end the results may be far more to her advantage than if she tries to shirk and looks only for what is easy and comfortable for herself.

It does not come within the scope of this work to point out the duties of the community at large with respect to the limitation of contagious diseases and the care of the sufferers themselves. The necessity for the establishment in every large city of a hospital especially devoted to the care of such patients has been insisted upon over and over again. Here I would only say that any nurse, who has contracted an infectious disease while engaged in the performance of the duties of her profession, has a right to demand proper care at the public expense and that such care can best and most economically be provided in special hospitals.

The personality of the individual woman is far more important and exerts a far greater influence in private nursing than in hospital work. So marked is this difference that, in the former, personal attractiveness — not mere prettiness, but the combination of externals and of qualities that make up a pleasing and attractive individuality — not infrequently goes for more than skill and devotion in the nursing itself. It is only natural that a stranger should at once form some general opinion of a nurse from her manner of dressing and her carriage, and that any sign of untidiness must undoubtedly create a bad impression.

While in the hospital, the nurse, when on duty, is always expected to wear her full uniform, and this, as a rule, may also be done in private families. But occasionally a nervous patient is apt to dread the sight of a trained nurse, since in her mind her presence indicates the existence of grave danger, and this dread is often intensified when she sees her in full uniform. At other times, the relatives may express a wish that the nurse should wear for a little while, or perhaps always, the ordinary dress of private life. Again, it is for many reasons inadvisable that a nurse should wear her uniform in the dining-rooms or about the corridors of an hotel. By so doing she not only makes herself conspicuous and may be subjected to the embarrassment of being rudely stared at, but also may cause unnecessary alarm to other guests. Her uniform makes it evident to those she meets that sickness is in their midst; or the rumor is very easily started, that the disease is contagious, and the danger is so exaggerated by timorous minds that many will leave the hotel in haste and thus cause a considerable, and wholly unnecessary, loss to the management.

When going to a private patient, then, a nurse should carry with her a good supply of uniforms, and a walking dress for use when she takes her recreation. If called to nurse in a hotel, she should also provide herself with some quiet, becoming house dress, that may be easily slipped on and off, in which to appear in the dining-room. Again, if the nurse has been engaged to attend an obstetrical case, and is obliged to wait some hours or days in the patient's house, the absence of the uniform makes her presence less conspicuous to the family and friends, and her every-day dress is apt to be more pleasant and comforting for the future patient, who does not need a constant reminder of what she has shortly to undergo. At other times, again, a nervous, capricious patient, while not objecting to the whole uniform, may take an intense dislike to some particular part of it, and may express a wish that certain modifications be made. In such instances, inasmuch as no vital principle is involved, the nurse shows good judgment in cheerfully adapting herself to circumstances, and in readily acquiescing with the wishes of those around her.

But if no objections are offered by others and the nurse is left to follow her own wishes in this matter, let her not hesitate to wear her uniform — the whole uniform as prescribed by her school and not a mutilated imitation. She should take pride in it as it is and not discard this or that part of it, or make alterations to suit her own ideas. She should not lay aside the cap, for fear that the wearing of it may detract from her dignity, because in bygone times it was a badge of servitude; nor should she substitute for it another which has been adopted by some other school, because she thinks it may be more becoming to her. A Yale graduate may regard crimson as a very handsome color, but he is hardly likely to wear a Harvard cap with the rest of his Yale costume. The wearing of the prescribed uniform does the nurse good by reminding her of her school, of which she must ever be a loyal and creditable representative; and at the same time it exerts a wholesome influence upon those around her. Unconsciously the patient feels that the wearer has a certain position of kindly authority over her, while, on the other hand, her uniform renders it more easy for the nurse to preserve the proper professional relations between herself, the physician and the members of the family. Moreover, I know of no other costume that seems quite so suitable for, or quite so attractive in, the sick-room as a clean wash dress with its accessories, the fresh white apron, collars, cuffs and cap. The light weight of the uniform also renders it more easy and comfortable to work in; it is readily put off and on; and it is always a comfort to know that one can go to one's next patient with everything one has on perfectly fresh, clean and dainty. So far, I know of only two objections which can be raised by the nurse to the wearing of her uniform — the expense and the difficulty encountered in a strange place in having it well laundried, for a cotton dress needs to be done up well, especially when the use of very little or no starch is insisted upon. But since the proper care of the uniform, as has been pointed out, is of no small importance, a few words with respect to this subject may not be out of place here.

The question of laundry arrangements is one that usually puzzles the young graduate. Some nurses expect the family to assume the responsibility of seeing that their laundry work is done for them, but this plan has never seemed to me to be a desirable one. In the first place, it seems more dignified to attend to these matters oneself; and secondly, at a time of illness, the laundry resources of the house are, as a rule, heavily taxed with the extra linen used about the patient and in incidental ways, so that it is manifestly unfair to put upon the housekeeper any extra cares. It is far better that, while in her own city, the nurse should arrange with a competent laundress to do her work regularly, so that she will never be obliged even to mention the subject of laundry in her patient's home. Even in a strange place she can easily make her own arrangements, although at times the results may not be all that she could wish. Again, when the nurse assumes the expense of her own laundry work, she is less apt to be tempted to be too reckless in the use of uniforms and personal linen, although of course, economy in this respect should never be carried too far, since cleanliness and daintiness are all important.

It is always advisable for a nurse, when she has made up her mind to do private duty, to supply herself with certain articles which she will need more or less constantly, and which she cannot expect to find in private houses. Of these the most important are a clinical thermometer, a medicine and minim glass, a hypodermic syringe, a Davidson or fountain syringe, and a pair of surgical scissors. A good supply of record sheets, temperature charts and a note-book for orders, should always be kept on hand, so that the nurse's reports may be started in a systematic way from the moment that she takes charge of a new patient.

Although it is not to be supposed that any large proportion of the many women who enter training schools for nurses are actuated solely by the desire to do good and are without any thought or consideration for the financial side of the question, nevertheless, in the ranks of trained nurses there are to be found not a few women who, being abundantly blessed with this world's goods, and being without duties which call upon them to remain at home, consider it a privilege to take their share in alleviating the suffering and misery around them without asking in return any pecuniary compensation. Far be it from me even for a moment to fail to appreciate the nobility of that spirit of self-sacrifice, which gives up ease and material comforts in exchange for a life of toil. And yet it must be remembered that, although they take no pay immediately, these women are supported by the institution to which they belongs and owe their food, clothing and lodging ultimately to the labor of others. In a word, since everyone, no matter how altruistic, must receive in return for his work at least a sufficiency for his daily sustenance, the question of remuneration becomes, after all, only one of degree.

From a consideration of the whole matter, it will readily be seen that no woman need hesitate to undertake nursing as a profession merely because she feels that her circumstances will not permit her to refuse all remuneration for her work. We have it on the highest authority that the laborer, even in spiritual fields, is worthy of his hire, and every one should feel it a duty not only not to become a burden upon others but to assist, perhaps in a pecuniary way, those who are unable to fight the battle of life unaided. It is clearly not only allowable but praiseworthy that a nurse should receive as compensation for her work not only a present livelihood for herself, and something additional to bestow on others, but that she should also be able to make provision for her old age, when she would otherwise have to depend upon the labor of others. Her nursing need not necessarily suffer because she receives pay for it. But on the other hand, if a woman sees in the profession of nursing merely a position which stands high with the public and in which she can make a competent living; if the pecuniary considerations are in her mind of primary importance, then all the beauty of the life is gone. If she cannot feel that she nurses for the sake of nursing, that she has something deeper than a mere liking for it, that she loves the work and takes delight and pleasure in it - as the true artist does in his painting - in a word, if the dominating principle in her mind be not to make her nursing help to mitigate suffering, to save life, restore health, prevent disease, and in this way contribute some small share in making the world better physically and morally — let her by all means choose some other honorable means of making a living.

But at the same time we should not be hypercritical or too ready to condemn the nurse who does not in the beginning have the highest ideals. I suppose that in choosing his career, every man is influenced by mixed motives, nor is he always conscious of the relative weight which his mind gives to each. I have no doubt that many a woman when she enters a training school for nurses, consciously or unconsciously, feels a good deal of satisfaction in knowing that she is practically provided for for the next two or three years, and that she is meanwhile receiving instruction which will enable her to hold her own in the world and earn an independent living. Nevertheless, I am happy to be able to say that, so far as my experience goes, the woman who does her work merely for the pay that she receives is a rarity in the ranks of trained nurses. Furthermore, it has often been a pleasure for me to note that many, in whom the commercial instinct seemed to be unpleasantly prominent when they entered the training school, as they gradually became more and more absorbed in their work and came to a fuller appreciation of its nature and responsibilities, also arrived at higher ideals and put material advantages in the background, where they justly belong.

The establishment of a scale of charges which would be suitable to every case presents many difficulties, since so many different circumstances have to be considered. In the first place it is desirable that as many of the sick as possible should have the best care, but relatively few families are able to expend a large sum for this purpose. At the same time, in the case of those who can afford it, work which requires skill and a long training and which is accompanied by a good deal of mental and physical strain, calls for no niggardly compensation. Again, all nurses do not give services of equal value, and a young graduate, fresh from the training school, would not in the nature of things deserve the same compensation as a nurse who has had years of experience, and who has been careful to profit by it and has kept abreast of the times. But although it is impossible to always adjust matters so that the services rendered may always receive exact compensation, some general standard can be adopted, the individual nurse being left free to make suitable modifications according to her own judgment and the necessities of the particular case.

In most places, then, we find that the rates vary between fifteen and twenty-five dollars a week and probably, as a rule, twenty-one dollars a week, or three dollars a day, can very properly be charged. When, however, a nurse feels that a family really cannot afford to pay this amount, but that the case is such as demands her care, she is perfectly justified in receiving a lower rate of remuneration. To meet these cases, it is better for several reasons that she should not adopt a sliding scale of charges, but make out her statement for the full amount at the regular rates and then take on as much as she thinks will be proper. This, however, should be done with tact, and the family should be made to feel that the diminution is, under the circumstances, an act of justice and that no favor is being conferred upon them. In this way the nurse will avoid doing injustice to her fellow-workers by lowering the prevailing charges for those who can afford to pay them, while at the same time the family will not think that they are getting any less than the best of nursing, simply because they are not paying the full rates.

On the other hand, the nurse is often called to take care of a patient, to whom money is no object, and under these circumstances she is justified in asking for the maximum rate. It happens, however, that not a few persons of great wealth are apt to think that they are being imposed upon, and at times a tactful explanation of the nurse's reasons for acting as she does — in one case receiving fifteen dollars a week, and in another twenty-five dollars for the same services — will be necessary in order to dispel this idea.

But no matter what is the rate of remuneration agreed upon, let the nurse see to it that her services are suited to the exigencies of the disease and are not regulated by the worldly means of the sufferer. Let her never put limits upon her vigilance and energy, in proportion to the lessened amount of money she receives. She may feel certain, however, that while in her mind pecuniary considerations are always kept in the background and are secondary to the work itself, it is only just and wise that she should receive her due, and that she need not allow those who are well able to pay for her services to take up her time without proper recompense, and thus prevent her from helping the poor and needy in their turn. Moreover, as has been said before, it is her duty not only to earn a sufficiency wherewith to support herself, but also to make provision for times of illness and her old age.

To the young graduate, who has never as yet earned her own living, twenty-one dollars a week may seem a goodly income, and she is apt at first to have extravagant ideas of her future pecuniary resources, and perhaps to act accordingly. But if she thinks for a moment, she will see that her total annual returns cannot be reckoned on this basis and that certain necessary expenses are going on all the time. During the year there will generally be a certain number of weeks during which she will have no engagements, but board and lodging must still be paid for, and an occasional vacation will also be necessary. From the very start, then, she should plan to live economically, but comfortably. She should never go beyond her income, and should always try to save something; above all she should never borrow; she should avoid extravagance in dress or the careless expenditure of money on little things that may catch her fancy, amusements, extra suppers or dinners, bonbons and trifles generally — unnecessary things, costing very little individually, but in the aggregate representing a greater expenditure than is required even for the necessaries of life. It is probable that nurses, as a class, are no worse in this respect than other women, but certainly thrift is not too common a virtue among them. I have heard it argued in extenuation of this failing that a life of confinement naturally leads to reaction, when once the nurse finds herself free. This has always seemed to me to be a weak excuse. Granted that private nursing entails a large measure of confinement, I know of no life of any worth that has not its own peculiar restrictions, and certainly my observation of nurses, who have done credit to themselves and their profession for years, has shown me that they have not found the demands made upon them by their work severe enough to compel them to discard all judgment as soon as the strain is over.

In her leisure time it is the duty of the nurse to take a thorough rest, combined with a sufficiency of healthy recreation, that will render her fitted mentally and physically to undertake the care of her next patient. Her health is all-important to her, for it is her capital and must be well looked after, if only for her own sake. Nor is it strictly honorable to go to a patient when half sick or tired out, for the strain upon the nerves is intensified and is injurious to the nurse, so that she is unable to give the best service. She should never be a valetudinarian, but she should be the last person in the world to neglect her health.

It sometimes happens, however, that while taking care of a patient the nurse will feel that she herself is not well; but provided she is sure that the indisposition is only temporary, she may continue her work. In any case it is never right for her to worry the patient with an account of her own ailments. But if she has any doubt about the matter, it is far better to quietly mention the fact to the attending physician and let him decide whether it is some simple condition which will soon pass off, or whether she is really prostrated from overwork or some serious sickness is threatening her. In the latter case, she must not persist in working, but should at once make arrangements to be relieved. This she must do, not only for her own sake, but because it would be unfair to add another sick person to be a burden to the household.

When in the hospital, matters have been so arranged for her that the nurse can readily carry out the ordinary rules for preserving her health; but when taking care of the sick in private families, difficulties will often be encountered. There may not be the same time or facilities for bathing; her sleep may be disturbed, her hours for rest and recreation may be cut short, so that at the end, although her health need not have suffered materially, she may feel tired and exhausted. Thus, as soon as the opportunity offers, she should devote especial attention to her personal needs, and her leisure time must be utilized for building herself up. For this reason she should always arrange to have comfortable quarters, either at home or in a house in which the surroundings are congenial. For the nurse who is a stranger in the city, the houses established by the alumnae associations offer exceptional advantages. Here she can obtain single meals or excellent board and lodging when at leisure, while at other times, when engaged in nursing a case, she feels she always has a place where she can occasionally drop in, when out for her daily walk, where she can meet other nurses and friends, and always find somebody who takes an interest in her welfare and in her work.

Let me warn the nurse never to try and cater for herself, or go to some cheap restaurant for her meals. To eat at irregular hours and to try and make out with poor food is false economy. Good, plain food, regular hours for sleep and a sufficiency of it, a bright cheerful room or home, a few congenial companions, as much fresh air and sunshine as possible, and a reasonable amount of amusement, are the best tonics for tired nerves and physical fatigue. A nurse should be the last person to spend money on drugs in the hope that they will make up for shortcomings in observing the laws of health. Moreover, in order not to get into a rut, it is always best for her to take a vacation of one or more weeks, according as finances will allow, and go right away from her work to some place where she will meet with different people and can enjoy a thorough change of scene.

A nurse need never have any spare hours which hang heavy on her hands. Besides devoting the proper time to rest and recreation, whenever the opportunity offers, she can attend alumnae meetings or lectures, which will help to keep her interest in nursing affairs alive and active. A certain amount of study should be arranged for, if possible — not enough to overtax the strength, but sufficient to furnish good food for thought and prevent her from falling behind the times. When waiting for a patient, the nurse should never give way to the inclination to spend her time in loitering or lolling about her room, doing nothing in particular. Good habits in the beginning are as easily formed as bad ones, and without them good spirits and good health are impossible. Above all, beware of forming the habit of self-pity; of always being sorry for yourself and bemoaning your lot; of looking out for slights and grievances, and finding fault with everything and everybody. When you reach that point, it is time to give up nursing, for you are unworthy of the work and incapable of meeting its responsibilities. Look for some other occupation in which, although such a spirit will never allow you to be happy, the indulgence in it will certainly do less harm. It seems to me that a good deal of the talk about the hard life of the trained nurse represents not only time wasted but a misconception of facts. Hard work, when properly met, after all, is seldom deleterious to health or happiness. How many women, who have nothing to do in life, fall victims to nervous prostration, and how few nurses, relatively, we find suffering from this disease. It has always seemed to me that the hardness of the life depends, to a large extent, upon the defects in the woman herself, and her lack of ability to adjust herself to surroundings and cheerfully make the best of everything. Given a woman of ordinary physique and a well-balanced mind, I cannot see any ground for the statement that a period of ten years is the limit during which a trained nurse can steadily continue her work. Much depends upon the individual; those less fitted for the profession, sooner or later, fall by the wayside, but at the present time I know many pioneers in the work, who are still actively engaged in it, and whose lives afford indisputable proof that the highest service may be rendered to humanity without any inevitable sacrifice of the health or true happiness of the workers themselves.

Chapter Twelve - The Case of the Patient

I have intentionally avoided devoting a separate section to the discussion of the care of the patient in the hospital, because I wished to emphasize the fact that the nursing for all patients — rich or poor, in the hospital or in their own houses — is in the main identical. Wherever she may be, the same fundamental principles should obtain, and the same spirit and motives should actuate the nurse in the performance of her duties. It is true that the accessories may differ, but where there is a deficiency of facilities, as happens in the houses of the poor, the nurse should supplement it by extra ingenuity and zeal; while an abundance of all the various materials, which render her work easier, should never make her less energetic or tempt her to rest on her oars. Thus I would have the pupil-nurse understand that from the first duty to which she is assigned in the hospital, from the first simple service which she is called upon to perform for some poor patient in the free ward, she begins the training which will fit her, after her graduation, to take care of the sufferers in the alley or the rich in their mansions. From the very outset let her determine that she will be no respecter of persons, but will treat all her patients with impartiality. While in the hospital, the nurse should always make it her rule to think of every patient— even the poorest and most unattractive — not as a mere case, interesting only from a scientific standpoint, but as an individual sick human-being, whose wishes, fancies and peculiarities call for all the consideration possible at her hands. If she has done this persistently, when she takes to private nursing, she will find little difficulty in adapting herself to her patient's requirements, while at the same time she will more readily recognize their various idiosyncrasies and will be the less likely to offend them or take offense. On the other hand, if the nurse has permitted herself to treat her patients as though they possessed no rights and were only just so many subjects being submitted to a given treatment, if she snubs them whenever they venture to express an opinion, arbitrarily overrules every wish, and in other ways shows that all things — even non-essentials — must be done exactly in her way, she is sure to meet her nemesis later on; for the habit by this time will have become so strong in her that, let her try as hard as she will, she cannot change her behavior at once, or before she has made for herself a reputation for being overbearing and dictatorial toward her private patients. In hospital work a woman of this disposition may occasionally escape criticism, since she may be clever enough to keep the head-nurse and the superintendent in ignorance of her true character, and the patients, from fear that their complaints will not be well received and that they will meet with even less pleasant treatment, or sometimes from a reluctance to be regarded as ungrateful or as chronic fault-finders, make the mistake of not reporting such behavior. As a rule, however, they take their revenge, after leaving, by talking against the hospital and the nursing staff as a whole, and doing their best to prevent their friends entering as patients or becoming contributors to the funds of the institution. If, however, a woman carries this habit with her into private nursing, she will soon suffer for it herself, as well as bring down sharp criticism upon her school. But leaving out any question of her own personal advantage, let the nurse resolve to start right from the very beginning. Let her resolve that her patients shall receive their due, or even more than their due, at her hands; and that through her presence, her' care and her thought, they shall be surrounded by everything that will hasten their recovery or lessen their suffering. If she could only remember to follow in every instance the golden rule of life — to do unto her patients even as she would have done unto herself or to one of her own loved ones in such a case — she would not be apt to commit many errors, and her ministrations would more nearly resemble those of Him, who pleased not Himself, but who came among men as a servant. The nearer to her heart she keeps the teachings and the life of Christ in her every-day work, the greater will be her strength to overcome difficulties and to forget herself in helping others. Let her determine, then, that the patient's wishes are always worthy of consideration, and that in all non-essentials they should be yielded to, even though they may antagonize her own. On the other hand, when the patient, through ignorance of the real state of affairs, or in the querulousness of sickness, desires something that is opposed to his best interests, it is the nurse's duty to be unyielding, although her authority should be exerted so pleasantly and with such tact and good judgment that neither the patient nor his friends feel that they are being thwarted, but that they are only doing right in following her suggestions.

All that has been said, in a preceding chapter, with regard to the nurse's personality has even greater weight in connection with private nursing. While she was a student in the hospital, she was never without occupation, for patients were assigned to her, who had little or nothing to say in the matter. But now she finds herself seeking a position for which there are usually other candidates, and she will be made to recognize the fact that a nurse is selected not for her technical skill or efficiency alone, but that personal attributes have no small weight with the physician, the patient and the relatives. Again, first impressions are sometimes all-important. Her manner of entering the room and her greeting, her ability or inability to overcome with ease the first little mutual embarrassment, and her quickness or slowness in seeing the first and best thing to do, may at the outset either strongly attract or repel the patient. The same habits of personal neatness should be observed; when on duty during the day, or when called up at any hour of the night, she should always be neatly dressed and with her hair in order. Frequent bathing, of course, is necessary, but discretion must be exercised as to the most seasonable time to be chosen, and the convenience of other members of the household must never be disregarded. Only recently a friend told me of a trained nurse who took her bath each morning while the daughter of the house prepared and served breakfast for the patient, who would otherwise have been obliged to wait until quite late for something to eat, after being awake from the early morning hours. In another instance, the two nurses both insisted upon the use of the bath-tub each morning, and sometimes in the evening, while the members of the family made shift as best they could. Can we blame these families for complaining that trained nurses are apt to be rather a burden than a comfort in the house of sickness?

The nurse should understand that everything about the room should be her care, and that the comfort and well-being of her patients, except when they are too sick to take much heed of externals, depend not wholly upon the actual nursing, but are also influenced in a large measure by the way these services are rendered, and by the attractiveness of their general surroundings. Many nurses seem to think that because they have all the day ahead of them, and because there is only one patient to be cared for, or perhaps two, where a baby is included, they have an unlimited time in which to do the necessary morning's work; and so, whereas in the hospital the patient would have been cared for and her room put in order in an hour or two at the longest, the nurse is sometimes found still at work at midday or even later. But despite the various hindrances which may be urged in excuse, such a condition of affairs must be looked upon as being wholly unnecessary, if the nurse is particular to carry into her private practice the method and system, which she has been taught to observe in the hospital. In this matter she should not be regulated by the patient, but should tactfully exercise a kindly authority. For the patient's sake, both for the moral effect and for her physical well-being, it is far better that things should be done systematically and on time. The nurse, who has had her rest broken at night, may think that she ought not to be expected to make a very early start in the morning. It is true that she may need sleep, but in any case the forenoon is the time for work, and only after that is done should the nurse consider herself free. She should be up by six or half past, in order to have sufficient time to make her own toilet, air her bedroom, arrange for her patient's breakfast and get her own; then come various little duties, such as arranging and freshening the flowers, seeing that a sufficiency of wood or coal is provided for the grate, and preparing any necessary solutions or dressings. In this way a good beginning for the day is made and everything is in readiness when the patient awakes, which she may usually be expected to do not later than half past seven, unless she has passed a restless night and has finally fallen asleep in the early morning. The room is now opened and aired, the patient being suitably covered meanwhile, after which, in winter, it is rendered of a comfortable temperature by an open fire or other heat. Next, the face and the hands of the patient are washed and her breakfast is given her. Even when this consists of only a glass of milk, these preliminaries should not be omitted and the nourishment should be brought to the bedside on a tray covered with a dainty white cloth. After she has taken her breakfast, the patient is allowed to rest quietly, while the nurse removes the tray with its contents, washes and puts away everything that has been used. Next comes any special treatment ordered, the patient's toilet for the day, the making of the bed, and finally a general tidying up of the room. All this will occupy the morning until about half past ten or eleven, when the physician's visit may usually be expected, so that he finds patient, nurse and room, looking fresh, neat, clean and ready to receive him without delay. After the visit is over and any orders requiring immediate attention have been carried out, the nurse gives her patient her nourishment and then arranges the light in the room so that she can settle down for a rest or nap. During this time the nurse occupies herself with preparations for her patient's dinner, in tidying up her bath-room and the place in which she keeps her extra supplies, in putting her own room in order, and in doing any extras that may need her attention. If there is a baby to be cared for, it may be bathed and nursed either before or after the mother's bath and then put down and left to sleep. This work, except under extraordinary circumstances, should not occupy the whole morning. After the patient has had her dinner, has been given any medicine ordered and has been made comfortable, the nurse is usually at liberty to leave her with some member of the family, while she herself takes a rest for an hour, or longer if necessary, or goes out for a walk. Before leaving the house, however, she should always give clear directions as to what is to be done for her patient during her absence, and fix a definite hour for her return. She must always come back punctually and in plenty of time to make the necessary arrangements for the evening meal. After this has been given, the nurse again leaves her patient in the care of some trustworthy person, while she herself utilizes the time in making her preparations for the night. At eight o'clock the patient's toilet is made, the room is aired, a glass of milk or some light nourishment is given, the light is lowered, and all is in readiness for the night. Even with a very ill patient, where work is almost incessant, order and method can be brought to bear and thus effect a great saving to the nurse herself, and preserve at all times the quiet and peacefulness of the sick-room.

As the patient progresses toward recovery, the arrangements should be gradually modified to suit the changed conditions, although the same observance of punctuality and method in carrying out orders, in giving medicines, taking temperatures, keeping records and making reports to the physician, must be strictly adhered to. Sometimes, particularly during the period of convalescence after a severe illness, there is a disposition on the part of the nurse to become a little slack, to overlook small, seemingly unimportant, orders; perhaps she may not take the temperature regularly, after it has been normal for some days, or does not give medicines punctually, or neglects to get the patient up or to put her to bed again at the prescribed time — little things, it may be, but which must always be done well by a conscientious nurse. Nor for her own sake should she ever give the patient or the relatives a chance of reminding her of a duty forgotten, however trivial it may be. Besides, human life is too precious to be jeopardized by slip-shod, half-hearted or indifferent methods and service, at any period of an illness.

The daily care of the patient's room should always be regarded by the nurse as one of her distinct duties, and she should take pleasure in leaving the mark of her training and personality upon it, by keeping it in all respects above criticism and making the details of her surroundings a source of pleasure to the patient. It should be allotted its separate amount of time and attention in the daily routine, and its own particular moments for a little extra care that will always keep it up to the mark and looking well. In the morning, with the opening of the blinds, should come the glance round and the few touches to make it presentable for breakfast. At this time, special attention should be paid to the fireplace, if there is an open fire in the room. As a rule, the nurse is not expected to clean out the grate and build a fresh fire, but if there is no one else to do it at the right time, she need not consider it a menial duty or as compromising her dignity. What she might be unwilling to do for well persons, she can and should do for the sick. During the day she should see that the hearth is kept brushed up neatly and the fire replenished. Again, she is rarely expected to carry up the wood or coal, but if occasion require it, the extra labor is not so great, for she can save up the daily papers, and when she goes down stairs for something else, she can take the opportunity for wrapping up a piece of coal of a suitable size in her newspaper, so that it will be ready for use when she needs it, with no trouble to anyone. So much depends upon the woman herself and her resources in all such little ways. The building of a grate-fire for instance, if done intelligently, is a matter of a few minutes to the nurse, and the quiet of the sick-room is not invaded, whereas the importation of an ignorant servant from the kitchen, with the necessary appliances, may require a great deal more effort and time, as well as much disturbance, to the patient, nurse and family. Also in the matter of saving her own footsteps and in making needless journeys up and down stairs, a little forethought will be of the greatest help. To carry down as many things as possible at one time, and to fetch up all the things she may need on her return, require only a little planning beforehand. While the patient is having her breakfast, if she is able to take it alone, the nurse may bring in the flowers and arrange them nicely. After the patient has been cared for and the bed made, the daily cleaning of the room is begun. In brushing up the floor, it is better to use a cloth tied over the broom; when the floor is bare, and the case is one of infectious disease, the cloth must be wrung out of a disinfectant solution. All particles of dust and dirt should be gathered up, wrapped in pieces of newspaper and either burned in the open grate or at once sent down from the sick-room to be put into the kitchen fire. It is always well to use a damp cloth for dusting any article that will not be injured by moisture. Everything should be handled daintily and deftly, so that it may not be damaged. Before starting in on a thorough house-cleaning of the room, which is occasionally necessary, it is advisable, if possible, to have the patient well covered up and rolled on a lounge into an adjoining room.

Particular attention should be paid to little things. Flowers, pictures and furniture should always be arranged attractively, and in such a way as to please the patient; the toilet stand should always look neat and orderly and no dust should ever appear on anything. All such trifles make up a large part of the life of the patient, in whose eyes molehills now appear as mountains, and who readily finds pleasure or annoyance in every detail of her surroundings. Above all, the sickroom should never be allowed to become the repository for all sorts of articles that are being used about the patient. Everything suggestive of illness — medicine bottles, glasses, spoons, syringes, bandages, basins, soiled towels, dusters, and vessels of all kinds — should always be kept out of sight. It is always best to have an adjoining room to use as one's work-shop, but when not even a bath-room is obtainable, as a last resource, a corner of the patient's room may be shut off by a screen, and the necessary clean articles may be kept there. In no case, however, should food be stored in the room; if no better place offers, milk, broths, etc., may be covered up and placed on the outside windowsill. The nurse should also be most particular that all vessels are kept scrupulously clean; after being used, they should never be allowed to stand about, but should be at once emptied, well washed out and scalded if possible. The lavatory and stationary basins should always be immaculate, and, when necessary, disinfectant solutions should be freely used. It seems incredible that women, who have had a course of training in a modern hospital and who have lived in homes with modem plumbing, should need to be warned of the danger of stopping up the drainage pipes by throwing refuse of all kinds down the closet, or any stationary basin. Unfortunately, over and over again, I have met with cases in which a multitude of heterogeneous articles — burnt matches, masses of hair, bits of cork, and even dressings — have been found choking the pipes, and the family have had to incur unnecessary expense for plumbers, as well as being exposed to the dangers which always belong to any interference with the sanitary arrangements of the house.

The conscientious nurse makes it a point to be careful in the smallest details and to do her work with as few demands and as little expenditure for supplies as possible. She should be a source of pure economy instead of extravagance to a family, not only by hastening the patient's recovery by her good nursing, but also by her ingenuity in saving them from unnecessary expense. Illness always causes a considerable outlay, which only the very wealthy can meet without having to curtail at some points. Appreciating this fact, the nurse should feel it one of her obligations to do all that lies in her power to, make this expense as light as possible without, of course, depriving her patient of any necessary appliances or comforts. Just here may be found a test of her resources and of her inventive faculty. To be able to use equivalents is economy and should be also a pleasure. She can exercise judgment in the matter of the linen, having relays of sheets and night-gowns that may be aired, instead of changed, and so make the laundry work lighter; she can use old ones, where it is probable that they will be stained; she can be careful with the various utensils or appliances, especially those made of rubber, not burning the bottoms of dishes, or breaking china or glassware; she need not be too lavish with alcohol, or dressings, or order her patient's food in unnecessarily large quantities. These are a few, among the many, ways in which a nurse may wisely economize.

Again, if she has acquired the habit of waiting upon herself she will be recognized as nothing but a help and never a hindrance in the family. Although she is there for a definite purpose and her obligations to her patient are pretty well understood, the very nature of her duties in caring for the sick brings her into such close relations with all the rest of the household arrangements, that sometimes she may hardly recognize where her strictly professional obligations end and another kind of service begins. On the other hand, families rarely know just how much they can expect the nurse to do and how much attention she herself will require. Apparently a few nurses have taken advantage of this uncertain state of mind on the part of the public, and have made too great demands in this respect, with the result that one is often told that nurses are too great a luxury, as they invariably require an extra servant to wait on them. That many people delight to exaggerate the faults of the trained nurse, I am ready to concede, but that such a statement is really applicable to certain, instances, I know from personal experience. In one house in which I was taking care of a patient, I noticed a young man stationed in the hall outside the bedroom door. At first his presence made no special impression upon me as I passed in and out, but finding him still there on the second morning I inquired the reason, and to my amusement was told he was there to wait upon me, since the former nurse had always expected to have an attendant. Besides being rigidly punctilious in the performance to the full of all her duties, connected directly or indirectly with the patient, the nurse should take a pride in doing necessary things for herself, and making her presence felt as a help and a sustaining influence in the family but never as a burden. Her duties can never be fully defined beforehand, even by herself, for they will differ with each patient; but they should always mean to her the performance of any manner of service that can in any way be of benefit or relief to her patient, or that will save life; nor should she waste her time in debating in every case whether this or that particular service comes under the head of nursing duties, or should be relegated to the servants. It is far better that she should occasionally do a little too much, and that her willingness should now and again be taken advantage of by mean people, than that she should miss rendering the many little services to others, which make the receiver happy and at the same 'time strengthen the character of the giver. Nor will a nurse, if she have any tact at all, be at a loss when it becomes necessary to take a firm stand and prevent herself from being imposed upon. One is frequently pleasantly surprised at the effect of such a personality upon the servants of the house, among whom, again, the trained nurse is popularly supposed to sow seeds of discord and unutterable trouble. The example of a nurse who goes quietly about her own duties, who never exacts attention as her right or requires to be waited upon, but who, on the other hand, is willing to render any little service; who can go into the kitchen and prepare a meal or some dainty for her patient, who seems to know intuitively where to find things for herself, and who always leaves everything she has used, clean and in their places, who is courteous and pleasant — not too distant, but never familiar — will generally make the servants vie with her in trying to be helpful to her in every way, and may even bring about a condition of harmony and content which may not always exist at other times. In exceptional cases, however, it may be impossible for the nurse to wait upon herself; when the patient is critically ill, and when it is impossible for her to leave the sick-room long enough to do things which would otherwise be among her regular duties, the nurse is justified in calling for extra help and having things done for her. In other instances, again, it will be impossible for a nurse to restrict herself to her absolute nursing duties, if only out of pure humanity; for instance, when the mother, or head of the household, is ill and everything is going to rack and ruin from the lack of any one who can guide or direct affairs, the trained nurse will deem it her duty and privilege to offer her help in things not directly connected with the sick-room. Here to do more than is written in the bond is simply a matter of duty and common Christianity and there should be no question of professional rights. Then, again, when the patient requires comparatively little attention, and time might bang heavy on her hands, or when there is a long interval of waiting, it should be a pleasure to the nurse to employ her hands in some useful work in the interest of her patient or the family, instead of doing nothing or spending all her time upon her own affairs. Such extra services need in no wise compromise her dignity or her professional standing, and should some people think that by acting in this way the nurse is lowering herself and accepting the position of a menial, they will not be long in recognizing that the spirit, in which it is done, stamps the character of the work, nor would any but the most selfish ever venture to presume upon so willing a service.

With the part of nursing that pertains directly to the patient there is much for the nurse to take note of, in order to successfully meet the various exigencies which she will encounter. Remembering that no two persons are alike, she will set herself to observe the special characteristics of every new patient, that she may be able to decide how she can best be dealt with. The first and all-important step is to gain the confidence of the patient, for as soon as she feels convinced that she is under the charge of a nurse, who is capable, and at the same time has her best interests at heart, she will to a large extent cease to worry and be hypercritical, and will willingly resign herself to what is to be done for her — a frame of mind which always tends to make the nursing easier and more effective. This confidence can be materially strengthened in the course of the first day or two, if the patient perceives that the authority exercised by the nurse is almost imperceptible and has nothing disagreeable about it; that she is not always being snubbed; that the amenities of life still receive due attention, and that her own ideas, wishes and suggestions are treated with proper respect; in other words, if she feels that her soul is still her own, and that she is not lying helpless in bed under the supervision and control of a task-mistress. To bring about this happy state of affairs, the nurse should constitute herself the patient's other self, as it were, she should take pains to familiarize herself with her habits, her tastes, fancies and temperament and then enter into a ready sympathy with them — a sympathy of a judicious kind that, while pleasing her, will be helpful and not harmful. Patients are not infrequently selfish and irritable, self-centered and expect a great deal. But it must be remembered that they are not always responsible for these defects; their early training may have been bad, and in any case, we cannot expect a perfectly healthy mind when the body is sick. Querulousness and irritability the nurse should regard as symptoms, indicative of physical disorder — as indeed in the majority of cases they really are — and if she makes up her mind always to treat them quite impersonally, she will often be saved a feeling of wounded pride, and the temptation to make some unkind retort. Again, this way of looking at things will prevent the existence of any strained relations between the patient and her nurse, so that the latter can go on calmly, as before, showing the same steady sympathy and forbearance and the same little thoughtful attentions, cheerfully gratifying any innocent whim, until the patient feels that in return she must be docile and not return evil for good. Be very watchful of the small comforts; regard them as so many useful medicines; the patient may not always realize that she needs them, but she generally appreciates them — the occasional changing and turning of the pillows or the freshening up of the bed generally, the proper adjustment of the light in the room, the bathing of the hot hands and face, or a hot-water bag applied to cold feet. But be careful that everything is done in the right way and at the right time; avoid a fussy activity, and never worry your patient.

In her over-anxiety to entertain a patient, a nurse is often liable to talk too much, and to forget that the times and seasons as well as the topics for conversation should be carefully selected. It is not wise to begin a long tale in the midst of the patient's toilet, or when she is being prepared for bed at night, and is probably sleepy. Besides, long stories at any time are apt either to be tiresome, or they may prove too much of a strain for the weakened nerves. The topics for conversation, also, are by no means indifferent; some subjects are too trivial, while it is clear that the choice of others is not only unwise but absolutely wrong, for various reasons. I am constrained to mention one or two here — not because nurses are ignorant of the facts, but because too often they appear to sin against knowledge. First of all, then, never speak of hospital experiences. To refrain from this is, I am aware, more easily said than done, for the strongest temptation generally comes from the patients themselves, who find nothing more delightful than to get the nurse started on hospital tales; they lead up to them in all sorts of ways, and are not put off with evasive replies. Perhaps the best way after all will be for the nurse to meet the issue frankly and say that hospital subjects are forbidden ground for her, except when discussed in the most general way. Again, patients love dearly to hear about others, not only those whom they may personally know, but even perfect strangers, and they try their best to get the nurse to talk about various patients and their families. But if the nurse finds that, despite the exercise of all her ingenuity she cannot turn the conversation to other subjects, it is better to say, once and for all, that she feels it a duty never to talk about her patients. At the time, it is true, the enquirer may feel somewhat annoyed and complain that the nurse is too punctilious; but in her heart of hearts she will confess that the loyalty, which refuses to discuss professional affairs and to deal in gossip, is highly to be commended; moreover, she feels greatly relieved on her own account and secretly respects the nurse the more.

Too great intimacy between patient and nurse is inadvisable and should never be encouraged. But when it happens that a patient, in her weakened state of health that has left her nerves beyond her control, has confided to the nurse secrets of her own or of others, these confidences should always be held sacred and inviolable; furthermore, the whole conduct of the nurse should be such as to assure the patient that her moments of weakness will never be blazoned abroad. Nor does this obligation to secrecy end with the period of professional services; none of the privacies of personal or domestic life, no infirmity of disposition or little flaw of character, observed while caring for a patient, should ever be divulged by the nurse, unless circumstances arise which render such a course an imperative duty. The same rule holds good also with respect to the actual bodily or mental ailments. Patients and their affairs should not be made a subject for conversation or discussion between nurses; silence is even more binding upon the nurse than upon the physician, inasmuch as the opportunities of the former for knowing her patient's affairs are generally far greater than those of the latter.

Thirdly, beware of being egoistic; do not talk about your own private affairs. Here, again, tact will often be necessary to parry many curious inquiries, although at other times the nurse may be filled with the desire to impress the patient with the importance of her family, as regards social distinction or intellectual qualities. I know of nothing more wearisome, even to a well person, than to have to sit and listen to eulogies on people she has never seen and in whom she has no possible interest. Better to be left in peace to die of one's disease than to be driven insane by thoughtless chatter.

But although the ethics of the sick-room, as well as common sense, are opposed to any form of gruesome talk and to all gossip, it is very necessary that a nurse should be able to talk pleasantly and intelligently at the proper time, and in this connection she will find a broad general knowledge and education of the greatest value. Friendliness and good-fellowship between patient and nurse should never be allowed to degenerate into a familiarity that allows of jokes which are not convenient, or crude personal criticisms, that soon do away with the mutual respect which should exist between them. It is rarely, if ever, advisable for the nurse to try and control her patients by means of sarcasm, or holding them up to ridicule in the eyes of their friends. Children in particular are very sensitive and are very liable to resent such treatment by sullenness and obstinacy.

In caring for a male patient, a strictly impersonal manner must always be maintained and nothing in the nurse's manner should ever betray either undue interest or any feeling of aversion. In ordinary, everyday life it is a man's part to show little attentions and courtesies to women, to do the fetching and carrying and waiting upon; and even when weak or ill, he may to a certain extent feel under the same obligations to attempt to show them to his nurse. But it must ever be remembered that, in these cases, the relations between them are strictly professional and must be kept on this footing, and that a nurse, who so far forgets her position and is silly and vain enough to accept such attentions, commits an act of grave disloyalty to her calling, shows poor judgment and takes a risk that is almost certain to result in unhappiness for herself. With all men, then, with whom she may be brought into contact, in the performance of her duties — physicians, members of her patient's family and the patients themselves — the nurse should make it an inviolable rule to maintain a courteous but strictly professional, impersonal attitude. Private duty has its own special temptations, and this is not the least of them; but if she meets them in the full purity and dignity of her womanhood, she need not fear that evil will ever befall her.

Another common test of the strength of her self-control and mental balance is afforded by the fulsome flattery and praise that is sometimes bestowed upon her. It is perhaps only natural that the friends of a patient, who has just passed through a critical illness, should shower unstinted praise and presents upon the nurse, who has worked so hard, and has helped so much to bring their loved one back to health, or that, for the time being at any rate, they think that there is nothing too good to be bestowed upon her and nothing too fine or good to be said about her. But lest she be puffed up by self-conceit and overrate the value of the services which she has rendered, let her reflect that an exaggerated gratitude may be short-lived; that to have done less than her best would have been culpable; that many others have done as well or better and that to meet such occasions we still have the command: "When ye have done all, say, 'we are unprofitable servants; we have done that which it was our duty to do.'"

There is also great danger that a nurse who has patients mainly from among only the very wealthy class, may be spoiled, inasmuch as she finds herself continually surrounded with luxuries, and many opportunities for pleasure and various forms of indulgence are open to her. A woman, who has not been on her guard and has not curbed any signs of self-indulgence as soon as they appeared, but has yielded to the temptation to have an easy, good time, may wake up one day to find that, what were formerly luxuries have now become necessities, and that to take care of a patient of strictly limited means is a hardship to her. The habit of self-indulgence is apt to grow, while the habit of being satisfied with any but the best work is weakened, until her increased demands and lessened capacity finally render her undesirable to physicians and to all classes of patients. The nature of a nurse's work requires good, nourishing, simple diet, but she may be tempted to allow herself a too liberal use of rich foods, when caring for a patient belonging to a wealthy family, and in this way not only upset her health but also form a habit of living luxuriously. Above all, let her make it a rule never to take a single glass of wine or any form of stimulant, at least while she is fulfilling an engagement. Let her settle this in her own mind once for all and let nothing make her swerve from her determination. The trained nurse occupies a position in which she is subjected to constant watching and criticism, and I know of no class of men or women who are expected to walk more circumspectly or more worthy of their vocation. Should this be a matter of surprise, when we consider that a mother is often expected to allow the care, the comfort, it may be the very life, of one who is dear to her and from whom she has never been separated, to pass out of her own keeping and into that of an entire stranger? Is it unnatural, that, at first at least, she should have a certain feeling of mistrust, or a kind of resentment against the nurse, as an interloper, or that she should treat her with some coolness and jealously watch her every action? Experience teaches that a patient does better as a rule in the hands of a good trained nurse than in those of a well-intentioned, but unskilled, friend or relative; and that in such cases love cannot take the place of educated intelligence. But the family cannot always be expected to realize this fact at once and, remembering this, it is the duty of the nurse to make every allowance for any coldness and any apparently unkind treatment that she may at first have to encounter. If she tries to imagine herself in the place of the relatives for the moment and forgets her own side entirely, she will probably decide that her behavior under similar circumstances would not be much better. Far from showing any surprise or taking any perceptible notice of a somewhat chilly reception, she will not resent it even in her own mind.

She sets to work at once to win the confidence of the patient and of the friends by her manner and actions; in a quiet unobtrusive way she makes things run smoothly, inside and outside of the sick-room; chaos, worry and excitement seem to disappear with her arrival; she adapts herself quietly to the ways of the family; she makes few demands for her own comfort; she devotes herself to the interests of her patient, although she is careful not to assert her full authority in the sick-room at first; gradually and almost imperceptibly the relatives awake to the fact that, after all, the ordeal has not been so very dreadful, and that no stranger, but rather a trusty and skilled friend, now has chief charge of their loved one. Moreover, only in comparatively rare instances will the physician consider it his duty to exclude from the sick-room all the relatives, and when the nurse finds that the wife, mother, or daughter, as the case may be, anxiously desires to share in the nursing, she can always make judicious use of their help. Frequently, when only one trained nurse can be procured, she has to select the most competent members of the family as her assistants, to work under her instructions, or to relieve her when off duty for her necessary rest or recreation. A skilled nurse, who does her work well and in a simple-hearted way, who is willing to put her own feelings and comfort in the background, will rarely fail to win the confidence of those around her; nay more, in a short time, far from being slighted or treated with coolness, she will be in imminent danger of receiving too much attention, which, however, must be tactfully turned aside. Her own aim, so far as the family are concerned, should be to deserve their confidence, to demand nothing unnecessary for her patient or for herself, to make as little extra work as possible, and as far as circumstances will permit, to provide for her own needs; to gladly and cheerfully render any little services outside the sick-room; always to give due consideration to any suggestions offered and give way to any wishes respecting her patient, when such a course would not be harmful. Not infrequently, indeed, the family may be of distinct assistance in the management of the patient, owing to their personal knowledge of her and of her likes and dislikes. The nurse should be on her guard at all times that no duty may escape her attention and that she may not need a reminder from some watchful friend of the patient. Where the family are inclined to interfere with her orders for her patient, it will be best for her to ask the doctor to write down the necessary instructions, or to insist upon them to the friends. She should always note carefully anything in the surroundings that may have a direct bearing upon her patient's condition, and should report it to the physician; but should any unpleasantness in the family life be apparent, she should be seemingly unconscious of it and keep her knowledge to herself. Nor should she be hypersensitive or too ready to take offence. In those rare instances, however, in which, despite her best efforts, the nurse finds after mature consideration that her temperament is incompatible with that of her patient or family, and that her presence is likely to be more harmful than beneficial, the wisest course for all concerned is for her to quietly resign her position, although she should not leave suddenly, in a moment of irritation, or until the continued care of the patient has been provided for.

It is possible that, while smarting under a sense of unfair treatment, the nurse may be tempted to talk about the family and their peculiarities; but no wrongdoing on the part of others relieves her from her obligation, never to make known anything which she may have learned about those with whom her profession has brought her in contact. While endeavoring always to maintain cordial relations with the various members of the family, the nurse should never forget that her position should always be a purely professional one; despite the fact that her length of service has resulted in the establishment of a mutual esteem, she should never fail to preserve the little invisible line of reserve, and be on the watch that her presence may never be in any way irksome or undesirable. For this reason, among others, one usually prefers to have one's meals alone, if such an arrangement can be made without any inconvenience to the family. The fact of being by oneself at these times, and free from an almost interminable series of questions about the patient, in itself is to a certain extent a relaxation, while at the same time the nurse can feel sure that she is not intruding upon the privacy of the family life at one of the few times that all the members have a chance to be together and to discuss purely family topics. In any case it is always better to have people wish that they could have seen more of you than to overstay your welcome.

Excepting during her hours of recreation a nurse's place is by the side or, at any rate, not far away from her patient. A proper amount of recreation and a regular change of air and scene are needful in the best interests of the patient as well as those of the nurse. In arranging for these, however, the latter should not try merely to suit her own convenience, but rather choose a time when some competent friend or member of the family can best arrange to take charge in her place. Again, the nurse should always look upon this time for recreation mainly as affording opportunities for building up, so that she can continue her work successfully, and for this reason she should not spend it in any way — such perhaps as shopping, attending to business affairs, or making formal calls — which would be more apt to tire than rest her. Make this also an unalterable rule. Never talk about your own little pains and aches with the patient or the members of the family. You are there to give, not to receive attention. When you feel uncertain about your health, consult a physician, and when he has decided that you are really ill and can go on no longer, make the necessary arrangements without any unnecessary words. A patient who is at all inclined to be selfish, is irritated by the complaints of her nurse; an unselfish one allows herself to be neglected, since she hesitates to demand the necessary attention from one whom she believes to be almost as sick as herself.

It is the wisest plan for the nurse not to expect to find her permanent friends among her patients or their families. Of course there may be the occasional exception to prove the rule, but generally speaking, with the termination of her professional relations with them, any efforts at keeping up an active friendship should also cease. To make an occasional call, at long intervals, to inquire for the patient's health, is quite proper, when one has the time; but to pay numerous visits will in most cases prove tiresome and inconvenient to people who have their own friends, society and engagements. For a nurse to accept an invitation to remain in a family after her engagement has ended, until another patient needs her services, is usually inadvisable. A business-like promptness in coming and going is more dignified and will, as a rule, prove more satisfactory to all parties concerned.

All things considered, the period of an illness that the nurse will probably find most trying is that of convalescence. We all understand the attraction that a good nurse finds in undertaking the care of a critical case of illness, that may mean days and nights of incessant work and watching, during which personal ease and comfort and even necessary rest are forgotten, the one thought and aim being to save the patient's life. But once the crisis is over and the imminent danger averted, there is naturally a reaction from the high tension. From the moment the patient is pronounced convalescent a different order of nursing begins and the nurse has to adapt herself to work which, while still sufficiently laborious and exacting, lacks the stimulus to which she has grown accustomed. One occasionally hears a nurse boast that it is her custom to nurse patients through the critical period of their illness and then leave them to the care of others. Such conduct — the willingness to desert a patient before the work is finished — is not only a serious breach of nursing ethics, but also shows a want of perseverance on the part of the nurse. Moreover, the level-headed, tireless woman, who is always ready to go through with any work she has undertaken, is likely to prove far more efficient in critical moments than one who cannot do good work unless she has the incentive of excitement to spur her on. As a matter of fact, convalescence, in order that it may end in complete recovery, requires its own careful nursing, and there is perhaps more credit due to the nurse who is a success at this time than to the one who did so well while imminent danger was threatening. To care for a patient who has become fully conscious of her surroundings and of her own weakness and suffering — if one desires to meet with difficulties — is no despicable task. At this time greater demands are made upon the nurse from the ethical side of her training and teaching, and her own personal resources are put to the severest test. Weary days and weeks have to be met, but whether they appear to the patient to be interminably long, or relatively short, will depend to a great extent upon the nurse. To the right kind of woman the situation is by no means without its distinct attractions; the patient is dependent for everything upon those about her, and a proper appreciation of the nature of the services to be rendered and the manner of rendering them is all-important. What may please and interest one may have the reverse effect upon another, and the nurse needs, therefore, to have a variety of resources at her command upon which to draw. The systematic planning of the day contributes not a little towards filling it with interest and lessening its tediousness. The patient has reached a point where she is more alive to what is going on about her, and each step in the day's proceedings may become a source of interest and pleasure or, on the other hand, of irritation; the judicious blending of necessary duties, of amusements and of rest, all appeal to her, and she unconsciously puts herself in harmony with them and thus hastens her own recovery, while forgetting the lapse of time. As her appetite begins to return, although she may not wish to know beforehand her menu for the day, she is interested in it when the time for a meal arrives, and is apt to enjoy her food in proportion to its attractiveness and the way in which it is served. It is not well to consult the patient in the morning as to what she would like to have to eat during the day. Notice when she expresses a preference for some particular dish and then quietly provide it for her at a time when she may be least expecting it. A variety in the kinds of food should be arranged for by the nurse, and if necessary, extra delicacies prepared with her own hands. Above all, everything should be daintily and attractively served. Little attentions to the patient's physical comfort before the food is brought, cleansing the mouth, smoothing the hair, sponging the hands and face, and shaking up and adjusting the pillows, are species of re-freshment in themselves and' add zest to the tray that follows, attractive in its fresh daintiness, in its little original touches and its unexpected surprises supplied by the contents of the dishes. The nurse should also be particular in her own handling of the china and of the food, always washing her hands be-fore either serving or cooking it, never using her handkerchief or touching her hair while engaged in feeding her patient, and never lifting cups, glasses, or bowls, by grasping the rim between her thumb and finger. The meal should be eaten leisurely and without haste, a pleasant interval being al-lowed between each separate course. As a result of the observance of these small amenities, the patient comes to look forward to the times for taking her nourishment as among the most pleasant in the day. The various ways of amusing or entertaining a patient can hardly be dwelt upon at this time; one thing should always be borne in mind, namely, that to do too much, and not to do enough, are equally objectionable. To obtain the happy mean, both when she herself is concerned and as regards others, frequently calls for the exercise of good judgment and an abundance of tact. The nurse has to main-tain a just authority as to the admission of friends and the length of their vis-its. Just here I should like to lay special emphasis upon the desirability of leaving friend and patient alone together. The old saying, "Two is company and three is a multitude," applies very well here, for a nurse is distinctly an undesirable element in the room at these times. Usually when a patient is well enough to see a friend, she is well enough to see her alone; the nurse may always place restrictions upon the time and keep within calling distance, but except in the rare instances in which her presence is required in the room, she should not remain, unless her patient particularly requests her to do so. Similarly, when a member of the family comes in for a chat, the nurse should quietly withdraw, after telling her patient that she will remain close by.

I have dwelt at some length upon some of the many faults and shortcomings for which the nurse may be severely criticized, and which she must avoid, if she would be successful in her work as a whole. Some of these may seem so trivial as to be unworthy of mention; some, I feel sure, will appear, to those who have not had a long experience, to be in the last degree improbable. As a matter of fact, I have been careful never to draw upon my imagination of what might possibly happen, but in every instance I have spoken only of things which have actually occurred — sometimes through the shortcomings of those who knew what was right, and of whom better things might have been expected.

To sum up briefly, the woman who would successfully carry on private nursing must put her work first and self in the background; she must add to a comprehensive practical ability, a strong attractive personality, that gives much and expects but little in return.

Relation of the Nurse to the Physician

It would seem as though the duties of the nurse as distinct from those of the physician, together with her professional relation towards him, should by this time be pretty generally understood; and yet at times certain misconceptions seem to crop up from both sides, with the result that the public also are liable to become confused on this subject. So far as the nurse is concerned, there is little excuse for any short-comings, since during long months of training in the hospital she has not only had careful instruction on these points, but has also had opportunities every day of appreciating the necessary distinctions and how this recognition should influence her own conduct. Unfortunately, here and there we find a nurse who, through ignorance — but far more often from the gradual growth in her of self-conceit and an exaggerated idea of her own importance — may overstep the boundary limit, and in her relations with the physician commit some breach of etiquette, for which not only she herself is made to suffer most acutely, but the school from which she comes and even the profession at large come in for a large share of blame and criticism. If then the nurse wishes to save herself a great deal of needless trouble in the future when she starts out to do private nursing, she will decide in her own mind that the physician is primarily and ultimately responsible for the life and health of the patient, and that it necessarily follows that the direction of the treatment belongs to him; and secondly, that the nurse, acting as his assistant, is bound to carry out this treatment loyally and faithfully without modifying it or changing it in any way. Moreover, if in prescribing the procedures to be employed the physician goes into minute details as to the way in which certain of them are to be carried out, his wishes are to be law to the nurse. The question whether she agrees perfectly with his recommendations, or believes that her own methods are better, has no bearing upon the case. Apart from the fact that she may be quite wrong in her opinions, her sole duty is to obey orders, and so long as she does this, she is not to be held responsible for untoward results. As a matter of fact, as she goes on with her work and gradually broadens out, she will recognize that there are more ways than one of accomplishing the same end well, although, when allowed to do as she pleases in regard to details, she will naturally prefer the methods which have been taught her during her training and which long practice enables her to carry out most skilfully. Moreover, in a few years, she will find that she has acquired a wider range of practical knowledge through these diversities of opinion and treatment. It is true, although almost incredible, that nurses have been known to expostulate with physicians, and to suggest that the treatment ordered was not best for the patient. I am well aware that, when this breach of etiquette has been committed, the nurse has often acted from a strict sense of duty, but besides the fact that "a good nurse is often a poor physician," and that she cannot reasonably be considered competent to judge of such matters, she can always remember that her responsibilities are limited. If a nurse has made up her mind that a physician is incapable, she can always find some means of refusing to take charge of the nursing of his patients, but once having put herself under him, let her remain loyal and carry out his orders to the letter. Nor is it honorable in the nurse ever to cast discredit in any way upon the physician, although she may sometimes be tempted to do so. The patient or some member of the family will often ask her whether things are being carried on exactly in the way that obtains in some given hospital and whether she thinks that any other methods would be better adapted to the case. It need hardly be mentioned that if the nurse sets herself up as a judge and makes any criticism, the only result will be that what she has said will be passed on to the physician and, without doing any possible good to the patient, the nurse herself will lose the respect and confidence both of the physician and the family. If, however, she is questioned by the relatives and she is really convinced in her own mind that in all probability the patient is not getting the right treatment, it is not for her to give her judgment of the matter. It is far better to tell the enquirers that, if they are not satisfied, it would be well for them to confer with the attending physician and then, if necessary, seek additional medical advice. So much needless worry and a great many searchings of heart will be saved to the nurse, who never fails to remember that she has been trained in nursing and has not received the education that fits her to assume the part of the physician. If she forgets this, she will at some time find to her cost that in medicine more than in anything else, a little knowledge is indeed a dangerous thing. In my own experience I have seen disloyalty to the physician, and a self-conceit that has led to forgetfulness of their own limitations, bring failure instead of success to nurses, whose knowledge and ability in their practical work was surpassed by few, but who by their behavior in these respects have stamped themselves as ignorant women, deficient in common sense and without any feeling of honor or honesty. Granted, even, that the physician in a given case may not be skilful — and on this point, I would insist again, the nurse is not always competent to judge — the responsibility for his engagement lies with the patient or his friends, and information as to his incompetency should never come from the nurse.

But it is not so much through any actual words of the nurse that she inspires the patient and friends with confidence in the physician; her manner, the way in which she receives his orders and her readiness in carrying them out, her professional attitude to him, always most respectful and attentive, never showing by the least sign any doubt in his ability, will be readily interpreted by anxious watchers. No matter how trying the occasion, a nurse should never show by her manner toward the doctor any shadow of rudeness, even although she may have but little respect for him or his ways. If for any cause she is obliged to oppose him, she should guard against doing so in the presence of a third person, but make her opportunity away from the patient's room. She should carefully avoid any criticisms of his methods, even if consulted on the subject. Some physicians allow nurses a great deal of freedom their work, rely upon their judgment to give certain medicines, when necessary, and upon their knowledge in emergencies or in the dressing of surgical wounds. But because this confidence is placed in her, she should be all the more careful not to overstep bounds and attempt a system of prescribing on her own account. Cordial relations cannot fail to be established between physician and nurse when the latter proves herself to be at every turn his faithful and loyal assistant, and he in his turn shows, by his manner and in other ways, his confidence in and respect for the nurse. If an opinion is asked the nurse regarding the relative merits of two physicians, she should frankly decline to pass judgment; she should never compare one physician's treatment with that of another; in fact she should remember that all such discussions are out of her province, except at such times as she is receiving instruction. Physicians are naturally irritated when they find that the nurse has been telling the patient or friends of the wonderful sayings and doings of her own pet doctor. Nor is it for the nurse even to make any suggestion as to the calling in of any particular physician, when a consultation has been decided upon. This is to be left entirely in the hands of the attending physician and the friends.

Again, not infrequently the patient or friends are so impressed by the nurse's skill and wisdom, that instead of consulting the doctor, they may come to her for advice about the ailments of some member of the family who may be feeling unwell. This insidious form of temptation, to assume the doctor's duties and to make a display of her knowledge, is constantly occurring, but any yielding to it constitutes a grave ethical offence committed against the doctor and society at large. Amateur doctors, as well as amateur nurses, sometimes do more harm than good. She should be most careful not to talk about or show off her technical knowledge before the patient or the friends, while, as regards the physician, she will best deserve his confidence by keeping strictly within her own limits, by watching for symptoms of any complications that may arise, by sending for him only when necessary, by her discretion in interpreting his orders with regard to medicines to be given in an emergency, and by keeping him in touch with all the facts relating to his patient; by carrying out his instructions accurately and punctually, by her well-kept, clearly expressed records and charts, which will obviate the necessity for any discussion of symptoms, treatment and results, in the presence of the patient. If any special features in the case have been noted by the nurse since the physician's last visit, she may make an opportunity for speaking to him about them outside of the sick-room, or she may draw his attention to the fact in a special note. At the close of the visit, after all the necessary orders have been given, the nurse may withdraw into the next room and leave the patient alone with her physician for a few minutes, in order to allow her an opportunity to say anything she wishes to him in private. In this way the nurse shows that she is more than willing that her patient should speak freely to her physician about any matters, which may not be to her taste, and that she still enjoys her freedom and is not under constant espionage. If left in charge of the patient after the physician's visits have ceased, the nurse should make reports to him at stated intervals about the progress of the case, thus providing a safeguard both to the physician and to herself in case of a relapse or change of condition in the patient later on. A careful attention to these and other details, which vary with different cases, will soon cause the physician to feel that in the trained nurse he has a loyal assistant and an active helper in bringing about the recovery of his patients.

It does not come within my province to speak of the obligations the physician owes to the trained nurse. Suffice it here to say that a kindly interest in her work and welfare, a readiness to aid her in every possible way, criticism made only in a friendly spirit, a certain amount of allowance for her shortcomings, a proper choice of time and place for reproving, when reproval is needed, and a show of such courteous consideration as shall increase the respect of the patient for her nurse, will rarely fail to evoke in return a more willing service and a more hearty co-operation. But if truth must be told, rare instances occur in which the physician is unworthy of the respect both of nurse and patient, and the former, when she has gone through one such unsatisfactory experience, is fully justified in avoiding the care of patients who are under his charge. Of course it is a mistake to be too sensitive or to take offence when none is meant, but although the nurse may be long suffering, so far as regards neglect of appreciation of her work, she is not expected to put up with unjust or rude behavior, and when she finds that, through no fault of hers and despite her best endeavors, she cannot work in harmony with the physician, she is fully justified in leaving the case as soon as an efficient substitute has been found to take her place. But no matter how great the provocation, the nurse must see to it that she is blameless in the way in which she protests against unfair or discourteous conduct. Thus, for instance, if the physician so far forgets himself as to speak harshly, or criticize her conduct or her nursing, in the presence of the patient, it is far more dignified for the nurse to keep her temper and not reply at the time; nor should she disturb the patient by any semblance of a scene or by leaving the room abruptly. It is far better to notify the physician by letter that he has rendered it impossible for her to continue the care of the case, and also tell the family her reason for wishing that another nurse should be provided as soon as possible.

Fortunately, such unpleasant occurrences are rare. Physicians as a rule are gentlemen and act accordingly; moreover, not a few of them are ready to appreciate the aid of a competent nurse and are glad to take her into their confidence and help her in every possible way. Thus, they can often make the nurse's task easier, by telling her beforehand about the nature of the case and of any peculiarities about the patient or the relatives, which might otherwise prove embarrassing. Above all, the honorable physician in his turn is always loyal to the nurse and by his manner will always show that he is convinced of her willingness and capability and will thus inspire the patient with confidence in her. In brief, harmony in the sick-room is indispensable, if the best results are to be obtained. Four factors — physician, nurse, patient and friends — must work as nearly as possible as one unit. Of the duties of three of these it is not my province to speak here — if discord should arise, let the nurse be careful that she is blameless in the matter.

But this obligation of loyalty must not only include the patient, the relatives and the physician, but must also be extended to fellow-nurses, not only of her own alumnae, but also those belonging to other schools and other countries — provided they are worthy of confidence. A nurse can give no stronger evidence of ignorance or narrow-mindedness than by behaving as if she considered herself, her school and her hospital better than any other. If she thinks for a moment, she will see that it would be not only impossible but highly undesirable to care ior all patients or to train all nurses in one hospital. Thus when two graduates from different schools are associated in the care of a patient, each should regard it as an opportunity to broaden herself and perhaps learn new methods in her work. Their professional relations should be marked by mutual courtesy, respect and good-fellowship; and no personal feelings should ever be permitted to interfere with their work. Any evidence of preference exhibited by the patient for one nurse over another not infrequently gives rise to many heart-burnings and bad feelings among the nurses. It sometimes happens that the nurse, who is called in later, may please the patient better than the one originally in charge, so that when the time comes for one of them to go, the second nurse may be invited to remain. Such an event, however, should never be resented by the one nurse, nor should it give cause for undue elation or self-satisfaction on the part of the other. With the next patient the decision may be exactly the opposite; in any case, it is the patient's privilege to choose, and any evidence of preference should be accepted gracefully by either nurse. Nothing should ever tempt one nurse to speak disloyally or criticize a colleague before either doctor or patient. If she is not all she might be as a nurse, let them find it out for themselves or through others. But, whenever a certain nurse has been known to commit acts likely to reflect upon other nurses or upon the profession, she should be dealt with privately by her colleagues as a body, and if, despite their kindly admonitions, she still persists in practicing irregular methods, she should be publicly dropped from the list of desirable nurses. The nurse may congratulate herself that such an unpleasant duty does not devolve upon her as an individual, but that, despite the absence of any legal restrictions to prevent ignorant or improperly trained women from posing as graduate nurses, the various alumnae associations are able to preserve the standards of the good schools by dropping undesirable members from their rolls and from their registers, thus making it evident to the public that these women, if engaged to take care of the sick, accept the duty without bringing with them any implied guarantee from the other members of good standing in the profession.

When two or more nurses are engaged to take care of a patient in a private family, it is the rule that the one who arrives first should take charge of the case, the second acting as her assistant. Such an assistant should faithfully obey all instructions, just as if she were acting under a head-nurse in a hospital. If, owing to temporary absence or illness, a nurse has been called upon to assume the duties of a colleague, upon the arrival or recovery of the other nurse, she should at once resign her position, since the patient does not really belong to her. Moreover, while acting for another, she should be careful, not to try and show her own superior methods by proceeding at once to make sweeping changes in the way of doing things; any necessary modifications being introduced gradually, so as not to attract attention. Nothing in the way of bad feeling, resentment or heated discussion, should ever be dreamed of; and not even a semblance of disagreement as regards methods should ever be shown in the presence of the patient. Since it takes two to make a quarrel, such an offence would justly call for the prompt dismissal of both nurses, inasmuch as at the best they have shown an unpardonable want of tact, and it is evident that unpleasant occurrences of this kind are impossible, when even one of the two possesses complete self-control. When one of the nurses is unworthy, the other has a hard task, but with tact and forbearance she will generally be able to finish the engagement without any apparent rupture. On the other hand, she is perfectly justified in refusing to be associated with the offender in the future.

Trained nurses are regarded by the public with very mixed feelings. As a class their position and the good they do in the hospital is now unquestioned, although, as was said before, individuals may be prejudiced against some particular nurse and her ways. But outside the hospital the trained nurse is still regarded as a not altogether unmixed blessing, and the public will need several more years of education — in which perhaps proper legislation, defining more precisely the standard requirements for members of the profession, will be of no little assistance — before they can be brought to thoroughly appreciate her position or the relative value of the services of the trained nurse and those of the untrained attendant or the well-meaning, enthusiastic, but untaught amateur. But meanwhile, there is much that every individual graduate can do in a quiet way to influence the tide of public opinion. Nor would it be reasonable for us to look upon legal registration or other legislative enactments as a panacea for the present unsatisfactory condition of affairs, for always, as now, it will largely rest with ourselves what status we and our work are to hold in the eyes of the public at large. The trained nurse, then, should teach those with whom she is brought into contact to expect of her the same high order of services, though of a different nature, as is demanded of the physician; and her instruction must take the form not of words but of thorough work and the most exemplary personal conduct. She should practically demonstrate to them that, apart from the fact that trained skill may be the means of saving life, when a cheap and incompetent attendant might fail through inexperience, the acceptance of her services, even when the highest fees are demanded, constitute a real economy, because, where there is intelligent and efficient nursing, many visits of the physician, which would otherwise be necessary, can be dispensed with; while at the same time far greater comfort to the patient is ensured, and his recovery is rendered much more rapid, with the result that the expenses of the illness are curtailed. Only after a long series of such results can men ever be expected to appreciate the fact that what is the best is always the cheapest in the long run. As an educator in the laws of health and right living, the nurse is gradually assuming her proper place, so that people are beginning to rely upon her co-operation to aid in preventing the spread of contagious diseases, by her timely precautions in places where she discovers their existence. By the way in which she does her work in the house in which sickness is present, she can teach the principles of home nursing and certain of the laws of health as regards proper clothing, the best methods of preparing food most suitable to the various conditions existing in health and disease, how to recognize certain adulterations of the more common articles of diet, how to guard against infectious disease, and how to meet emergencies. As a profession, as time goes on, we shall more and more be called upon to arrange organized nursing forces with which to aid in meeting any great public calamity or violent epidemic of disease, while at the same time each individual nurse is expected to do her share on all occasions where her presence is required, even at any risk to her own life.

Such are some of the responsibilities towards the public which every graduate takes upon herself — responsibilities which call for a special fitness to be supplemented by a special training. And after years of toil, after nurses, as individuals and as a united profession, have shown themselves to be necessary for the public welfare, it will most assuredly come about that, more and more, people will come to the conclusion that capability in nursing does not come by chance, and that a natural liking must be supplemented by education and practical training; they will gradually appreciate the fact that a trained nurse has spent time, money and much physical effort, in acquiring her education, that the mental and physical strain is more arduous than that belonging to any other kind of work done by women, and therefore, that this expenditure deserves suitable recognition at their hands. The friends of the sick will understand that the nurse takes charge of a succession of patients, not only one in a life-time, so that if she exhausts all her latent energies on their dear one by devoting herself day and night to caring for him without proper rest, food and exercise, she will be in no possible condition to go on to some other sufferer and do equally well; if she makes the attempt too often, she finally ends in breaking down physically, so as to be obliged to discontinue her work, and the public loses the services of a valuably servant through its own selfishness and thoughtlessness in overtaxing her. Moreover, as time goes on, those who were ever ready to criticize her efforts and to treat her as an interloper, will gradually learn that the world is better and happier from her presence, and that absolute perfection and flawless work should not be demanded at all times from nurses while they remain mere human beings. On the other hand, those friends, whose appreciation has often been shown by a not always wise enthusiasm, may come to appreciate the fact that the best of us are liable to have their heads turned by exaggerated praise and too much adulation. Nor will her name always be associated with sickness only, for in a majority of the movements for the betterment of the masses, the training of the nurse will fit her to take a useful share.

It is only by utilizing all the means at our disposal and by a steady application, which is ever seeking to add to our known resources others which are gradually being developed; above all, it is only by doing our work for the work's sake, that we can have to obtain the best and the most far-reaching results, and that our chosen profession will stand out as a beacon, ever kept bright by the light of our choicest personal endeavors, that will cause it to shine with a penetrating and attractive light, towards which all, who when in physical and mental suffering need to be ministered unto, may turn with the full assurance that they will not do so in vain.

www.ingramcontent.com/pod-product-compliance
Lightning Source LLC
Chambersburg PA
CBHW032008190326
41520CB00007B/402